# FUEL YOUR RIDE

# FUEL YOUR RIDE

## COMPLETE PERFORMANCE NUTRITION *for* CYCLISTS

**MOLLY HURFORD**

with **Nanci Guest, MSc, RD, CSCS**

RODALE.

## RODALE *wellness*

*Live happy. Be healthy. Get inspired.*

Sign up today to get exclusive access to our authors, exclusive bonuses, and the most authoritative, useful, and cutting-edge information on health, wellness, fitness, and living your life to the fullest.

**Visit us online at RodaleWellness.com**

**Join us at RodaleWellness.com/Join**

Rodale books may be purchased for business or promotional use or for special sales. For information, please write to: Special Markets Department, Rodale Inc., 733 Third Avenue, New York, NY 10017

Printed in the United States of America
Rodale Inc. makes every effort to use acid-free ∞, recycled paper ♺.

Photos by Ethan Glading—pages xix, 13, 54, 58, 63, 64, 92, 107, 117, 135, 136 & 157

Photos by Molly Hurford—pages x, 3, 22, 41, 100, 102, 104, 108, 115, 119 & 122

Illustration by Molly Hurford—page 49

Book design by Christina Gaugler

Library of Congress Cataloging-in-Publication Data is on file with the publisher.

ISBN 978-1-62336-619-3 paperback

Distributed to the trade by Macmillan

2  4  6  8  10  9  7  5  3  1  paperback

## RODALE.

Follow us @RodaleBooks on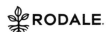

We inspire and enable people to improve their lives and the world around them.

rodalewellness.com

To the rad people in my life
who put up with the insanity of living with a writer,
especially those who submitted to being
interviewed for this book.

# CONTENTS

# INTRODUCTION

Chicken wings dripping with blue cheese dressing. A massive pile of fries. A thick milkshake—vanilla and peanut butter—to wash it all down. The beauty of it was, I was eating healthy. At least, in my head I was. After all, I was a vegan cyclist, so didn't that automatically make me superior to the omnivore cyclists out there?

Of course, I was a vegan eating fake chicken wings and a fake milkshake at a vegan fast-food joint in New York, which was rumored to have fought the city's ban on trans fats, because it's what made most of the food taste so good. Well, that and a lot of chemical processing, sugar, and nonanimal-product-based fat. But still—I'd read plenty of books on how eating vegan was the only way to truly be healthy, and since I wasn't eating any animal products, I assumed that I was in tip-top shape.

Fifteen pounds and elevated blood pressure later, I finally made the connection. It wasn't that I wasn't training hard enough—my racing was going great, and I was putting in massive hours on the bike every week. It was that, despite the trappings of a vegan diet, I was eating like crap. And my training could get a whole lot better if I just looked at my diet with a critical eye.

Our brains can rationalize a great deal, for instance, that huge cookie after a 90-minute easy ride, those two bagels mid–century ride, that energy gel while spinning 20 minutes to work. For me, it wasn't the vegan diet that was bad, per se. It was that I had started to find loopholes to avoid healthy eating while still sticking to a diet that I had heard was so good for me.

I was training 20 hours a week at the time, and it was easy to convince myself that an entire pizza (topped with french fries, not cheese—it's vegan that way) was a reasonable dinner. When I was riding, though, I was a food rock star. I had my hydration down to a science; I was skilled at drinking on the bike; and I was adept at eating gels on an hourly basis almost instinctively. But what I didn't realize at the time was that my nutrition off the bike was impacting my performance on the bike.

You can't start nutrition when you start pedaling. It's already too late. As nearly every dietitian and pro racer I interviewed told me, over and over and in several different ways, nutrition before the ride—hours, days, weeks, and months before the ride—matters more than what you eat during the ride.

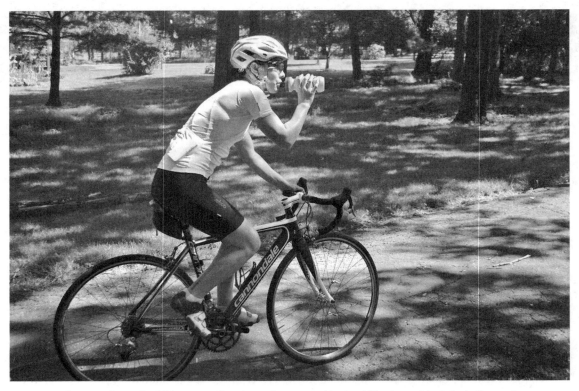

Once you're on the bike, you can't make up for a year of bad nutrition by suddenly hydrating and fueling right. Nutrition starts long before your ride begins.

My vegan diet had turned into a high-carb, high-sugar, high-crap diet. It was enough to keep me moving, but not enough to keep me particularly healthy, or happy. It's not that vegans can't be great athletes—just ask retired pro cyclocrosser Mo Bruno Roy—but when you live by the rules of the diet with no regard to what's healthy or smart, you get into trouble fast. And that's where I was.

Problems start to happen when you focus more on the diet than what your body is telling you and common sense. That's where this book comes in. While eating sensibly—more vegetables, fewer soft drinks, and a good mix of protein, fat, and carbohydrates—seems obvious for most of us, it's harder to execute in practice, especially if we're putting in big hours on the bike and we're just plain hungry.

It's difficult to determine the absolute best nutrition for a cyclist. There are plenty of fad diets, plenty of weight-loss diets, and plenty of hype out there. Research shows one thing, your buddy says another, your dietitian disagrees, and yet another study conflicts with the first one! So, what is a good diet for a cyclist? How do you get lean while staying strong, and how do you prepare for a long ride, or a hard effort, without sabotaging your weight-loss goals?

Pro cyclists are admittedly crazy about weird diets, and retired pro road racer Ted King is no exception: Over his years as a pro, including being one of the few Americans to race in the Tour de France, he's tried a multitude of trendy diets. Ask any of the pros who've managed to make a true living out of racing, and you will see that a balanced, whole-foods-based approach is something that they all have in common. "I've done the Paleo diet, I've done the gluten-free diet, I've done living like a monk," King admits. "I've done all of these things. I've been racing professionally for a decade. You learn one heck of a lot over your own experience, and then through watching other people's experiences."

King has developed his own new nutritional philosophy, and it's one that's really in line with what we will talk about in this book. "I think there is something to be said about 'ride to eat, eat to ride,'" he explains. "You know, there's enough head cases in the sport already, as there are in any professional sport, and so it's very easy to get tripped up in so many philosophies. You can eat Paleo, you can eat gluten-free, you can eat super-traditional cycling style—pasta everything, bread everything. You can subscribe to this or that or whatever nutritional guideline."

The diet's name isn't the point; rather, it's what goes into your body. Paleo is only good until you've pounded beef jerky and you have heartburn, and gluten-free is only healthy before you start chowing down on that tray of gluten-free brownies. "You spew through so many calories on the bike and you have to refill them, but maybe the philosophy should be 'eat to ride, ride to eat . . . with a wholesome and healthy outlook,'" King says, expounding on his original philosophy. "So you can't be eating doughnuts all day, but it's a privilege to be able to eat as much food as we really have to."

Most diet books are written by one expert, and while they often make a few great points, they often suffer from a professional or personal bias. This book, on the other hand, looks to several nutritionists—both researchers and practitioners—as well as the actual pro cyclists that we as riders strive to emulate. It considers the best research available—not just the newest info but also the most well documented from the past—and puts together a clear approach to healthy eating for the active, busy cyclist, both on and off the bike.

In this book, you'll find not only information about how and when to eat but also explanations of why you should eat this way. Why should you eat a protein-dense breakfast when you have an afternoon workout versus a carb-heavy breakfast when you have a 9:00 a.m. spin class? Why should you search for an in-ride food that has a bit of protein and fat for a century, but reach for a carb-only gel when doing a 90-minute interval training session? And perhaps most important, how do you make 11-time U.S. Cyclocross National Champion Katie Compton's super-top-secret gluten-free chocolate chip cookies?

We will explore the macro- and micronutrients that are important to a cyclist's diet, identify the best food sources to find them in, and then teach you how to incorporate those ingredients into super-yummy ride snacks. It's not enough to tell you how to eat, you also need to understand why certain foods are better at certain times, so you can tailor a diet that best suits your needs. A cyclist training 10 hours a week and working 9 to 5 in an office has different lunchtime needs than a night-shift worker who rides 6 hours a week, and both of those are different from a stay-at-home dad who rides 12 hours a week with kids in tow. That said, there are certain rules and ways of eating that can help all three of these people ride stronger, but each person needs to learn how to apply and adjust the rules according to their lifestyle.

And speaking of rules, another problem in the nutrition industry—with fad diets and uninformed nutrition bloggers spreading misinformation—is that while most of us think we know plenty about nutrition, we really don't have all the facts. One myth that Nanci Guest, MSc, RD, CSCS, loves to cite is, "You learn that a pound of muscle burns 50 extra calories per day, but that just isn't the case. It's actually closer to 11 to 13 calories." Does that mean you don't want lean muscle? Not at all. But it does mean that you might be counting calories inaccurately, or tricking yourself into thinking that your midnight snack will work itself off.

Myths come and go: In the eighties, we were told that fat was the devil and needed to be exorcised from our diets, which gave rise to low-fat and no-fat alternatives of our favorite foods, which were stuffed to the gills with sugar to improve taste. It turns out fat is a pretty important ingredient when it comes to making things delicious.

Fast-forward to current day, where we are hearing tons about how sugar is the reason for our obesity epidemic and a high-fat/low- or no-carb diet is the only solution. Again, we're hearing what we want to hear. We need an enemy that we can control, and when bacon can be in every meal, this carbs-are-the-enemy situation sounds pretty darn doable.

But, as Guest explains, "It's not as simple as low fat being to blame. People are eating more, and eating more junk." It's not about one specific food group, and demonizing a single macronutrient isn't the answer. While there is a problem with sugar and fat, the main issue is eating too much of it and not getting enough activity to support that high intake. On top of that, the excess calories in junk carbs, which are packed with both fat and sugar (think doughnuts and milk chocolate), are lacking nutrient density. We only have so many calories per day, so why waste them on garbage, whether it's saturated fats or white sugar and junk carbs like doughnuts, soda, and candy.

"Anytime you're getting into extremes, it's usually a problem," Guest says. "And the people behind the ideas, people who are so strong in these opinions, the more extreme and the louder they are, the less they know. Because they're not as open to new research that goes against their beliefs. If someone showed me that a higher-fat diet was right for athletes, if I saw that in the research, I'd change my mind. But the evidence just isn't there, and I'm not changing my mind to what's popular: I'm a scientist."

It's not just the kooky diet bloggers out there causing an uproar—the science community is equally perplexed, and new studies are coming out every day that seem to contradict prior works. If you think that sounds confusing, that's because it is. "There's a lot of transition right now, and we're going to find out even more in the next couple of years," Guest says. As a researcher at the University of Toronto working with high-level athletes, she sees all of the new studies being done and admits that the answers are rarely black-and-white.

The science is actually starting to shift toward a new, highly individualized paradigm. With studies looking at the different ways our genes influence everything from how we metabolize different types of foods to how we can best fuel our training, it's a brave, new world, and it's hard to say exactly what combination of foods is right for any one person.

Nevertheless, whole foods and a balanced diet—with a few tweaks that we'll get into later—is generally a good bet. "For the average cyclist not looking to make those tiny gains that the pros are working to eke out of their diets, the research that already exists is plenty to go on," Guest says. "If you're not trying to be a world champion, we have 99 percent of the information that you'll ever need."

And still, a lot of people run into brick walls. Not just weight-loss plateaus or performance-related plateaus. Mental plateaus are the hardest problem to overcome. "A lot of people try a specific approach; for example, they try to go low carb, and then they go low carb harder when that isn't working," Guest explains. "But maybe you actually need to change to get results. If you're doing the same thing and not getting results, you need to change it up. We're all very individual, so what works for one person may not work for another. It's a bit of trial and error." It's a good idea to tinker with individual diets to find out what works for you—not your ride buddy.

I believe in the idea of simplicity in all things diet related—I have to, for my own sake. Otherwise, I'd be back to eating vegan cheesecake and calling it health food. That, or I'd be sitting in the middle of my kitchen, food splattered and in tears because a recipe I was trying had gone horribly awry. From function (recipes) to ideas (fad diets), I believe that most people respond best to simple, easy-to-follow recipes and advice. I'm an impatient cook at the best of times, and I'm willing to bet that most of you are, too. So instead of complicated things like a 20-ingredient recipe for a gluten-free pancake, I'll showcase a recipe that involves just sweet potatoes, eggs, and a bit of cinnamon with maple syrup. I don't want you to spend a fortune to eat well, and while you'll see a lot of staples that pros and nutritionists swear by in this book, none of them will be mail-order only.

I don't have a diet agenda, other than a return to sanity.

No one person has all the answers, and I don't pretend to. So in this book, I'm not alone.

I've read countless studies, and you'll hear about those, but you'll also hear from a variety of nutrition experts with thousands of hours of practical experience working with cyclists. I'm working with several reputable experts, from nutritionists to pro racers, and I think that this approach—this willingness to take advice from other experts—will produce a balanced approach to cycling nutrition. We can't be right all of the time, but if we all agree on certain points, you know we're on to something. And that something is good, solid, easy-to-follow nutritional advice.

Before we get going, I'd like to offer a quick comment about this book. If you're looking for a book packed with dull graphs, charts, and diagrams, this isn't it. My goal is to present a healthy diet—not one that you'll keep for one virtuous month a year as you pick back up with your spring training—but rather, as a lifestyle that you can read, learn from, and use as you go into the grocery store, as you plan out your dinner, and as you pack your food for your ride and fill your water bottles. Don't panic: There are still plenty of calculations, numbers, and serious research in the following pages; the information is just presented in a different way than you've seen in nutrition books in the past. This book is for readers who need that nudge in the right direction but balk at the idea of being told exactly what to eat. It's for readers who are willing to experiment with their diets. It's for readers who know that, as individuals, their needs may differ from those of their riding buddies, and that's okay. We're all different, and there isn't one right answer when it comes to nutrition. There are, however, a few basic principles that we can understand, implement, and tweak to best serve our goals.

# SOME OF THE NAMES YOU'LL SEE IN THIS BOOK

**Nanci Guest, MSc, RD, CSCS:** When I first met Guest, I had a serious bone to pick with her. My boyfriend was avoiding caffeine at the time, and it was all her fault. Actually, he was participating in one of her studies as she worked toward her PhD—she was running a study to see how genetics modifies an athlete's response to caffeine under various exercise conditions and what genotype makes you a responder versus a nonresponder. That meant that there was no longer coffee—or even black tea—in our apartment. I cursed her name as I snuck out early in the mornings for my caffeine fix.

But once the study was over and we officially met (while I still held a bit of a grudge), I couldn't deny our shared view of simple and whole-foods-nutrition for endurance athleticism. And so, Guest became my primary expert, and the one you'll hear the most from during the course of this book. She became a great friend as well, especially after I learned that she thinks coffee is just fine. She's not just a talking head. In addition to a whole slew of fancy initials after her name, she has practical experience as well, from personal training to serving as lead dietitian for both the 2010 Winter Olympic Games in Vancouver and the 2015 Pan American and Parapan American Games in Toronto.

Guest is a registered dietitian with the College of Dietitians of both Ontario and British Columbia. She's a certified personal trainer and certified strength and conditioning specialist with the National Strength and Conditioning Association. Her main focus is the concept of highly individualized nutrition and teaching clients how to find what's right for each of them, which aligns perfectly with my philosophy of clean eating and finding the best approach for an individual.

**Jordan Dubé:** Dubé is the staff nutritionist for the Cycle-Smart coaching program in Massachusetts, and she has tons of hands-on experience working with cyclists and their specific needs. She says, "I think of myself as a diet therapist more than a nutritionist," because she prefers a more one-on-one dialogue with the athletes she works with, compared to handing over a one-size-fits-all eating plan. Her principle—that it's essential to learn what works for you within the general guidelines of a healthy whole-foods-based diet—fit perfectly in this book. "Balancing your diet with real foods is really all there is to it," she says. "I'm not super-scientific about it, I'm talking to real people, not scientists. I'm talking to real people who need me to tell them to eat real food and make them accountable for their eating."

**Peter Glassford:** Glassford is one of the few cycling coaches I know that really tackles—intelligently—all aspects of cycling, from knowing how your muscles move off the bike, to teaching incredible bike skill work, to suggesting basic nutrition guidelines to clients. Glassford runs Smart Athlete, a coaching company based in Ontario, Canada, and, as a long-time elite cyclist with a degree in kinesiology, he has movement down to a—pardon the pun—science. He chimes in on some of the more practical elements of an athlete's diet (i.e., you can't drink enough water in-ride if you don't know how to get the bottle out of the cage) to the more esoteric and downright philosophical question of what makes a cyclist's body so unique.

**Alexa McDonald, RD, CDN:** McDonald is a registered dietitian and certified dietitian nutritionist throughout the New York and New Jersey metropolitan areas. As an avid runner, McDonald's personal and professional focus remains on sports nutrition as she continues to work toward becoming certified as a specialist in sports dietetics. McDonald grew up in West Chester, Pennsylvania, and currently lives in Hoboken, New Jersey, where she works as a registered dietitian specializing in sports nutrition, eating disorders, weight management, and food allergies.

**Stacy Sims, MSc, PhD:** Dr. Sims is a well-known expert when it comes to the physiological differences between men and women. She's the chief research officer and former cofounder of Osmo Nutrition. As an exercise physiologist and nutrition scientist with 2 decades in the field (and an athlete in her own right), Dr. Sims was exactly who I wanted to talk to when it came to women-specific needs and in-exercise hydration.

**Jeanne Walsh Smith, RDN, LDN, RYT:** Smith is a registered and licensed dietitian nutritionist, registered yoga teacher, and the owner of Lehigh Valley Nutrition. Her clients include both large corporations and individuals interested in sports nutrition, weight management, and healthy childhood eating. With a lifelong interest in sports and exercise, she is also a registered yoga teacher, and stays active in Easton, Pennsylvania, with her husband and three children.

And then, there are the pro racers. After all, you're reading this book because you want to be an athlete, so why not look at what some of the best in the field are doing? The thing is, they aren't all doing the exact same thing. And that's great, because they shouldn't be: They aren't all the same—as racers, as people, or as organisms digesting other organisms.

**Katie Compton:** Compton has won every U.S. National Cyclocross Championship in the past 11 years—she's one of the best cyclocross racers in the world and has found herself on the podium for elite women at countless World Cups and even World Championships. Compton is one of the pickier athletes I interviewed, opting for a gluten-free antihistamine diet, yet somehow, most of her nutritional philosophies still line up perfectly with the other pros. Just because a truly world-class athlete opts to eliminate certain foods, basic principles of a healthy diet stay the same.

**Georgia Gould:** Gould is a pro mountain biker, but with a twist—she is a trained chef! So when you talk about a woman who's on top of her nutrition, Gould is the one to talk to . . . especially if you need cooking tips. She eats anything from kale to cupcakes and has uttered the phrase, "If it means no sugar and you win the gold medal at the Olympics, then maybe the gold medal isn't for me." That didn't stop her from scoring a bronze medal at the 2012 Olympics in London, so clearly the cupcakes aren't hurting her. Her background as a chef has made it easier for her to eat at home, make delicious meals from whatever is in her cabinets, and use all sorts of fruits, veggies, and meats in different ways to keep variety in her diet even when the ingredients are simple.

**Janel Holcomb:** Holcomb's favorite story to tell is about visiting her parents and having them stock the fridge for her weeklong stay, only to finish the fruits and veggies that her parents believed would last a week in the first 24 hours. As a pro road racer who rides long hours, Holcomb loves food—a lot—and her favorite part of riding is that she has the ability to eat what she wants. She primarily eats fruits and veggies, but nothing is off-limits,

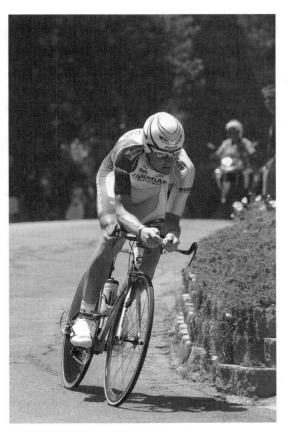

Retired pro road racer Ted King loves riding, but he loves food—especially salads—just as much.

and she admits that she actually has a specific chocolate drawer in her refrigerator. Fantastic!

**Ted King:** King retired at the end of the 2015 season after having been a pro roadie with Cannondale for 9 years. He's been on the pro tour circuit for the past 5 years, and yes, he's raced in the Tour de France. He's also an entrepreneur. When the whole-foods craze hit cycling, the pro peloton was divided between those eating rice cakes and those still sucking down gel packs of processed sugars. King, being a native Vermonter, wanted to inject some whole-foods quality into a gel pack and helped start UnTapped—gel packs filled with pure Vermont maple syrup. Talk about the best of both worlds! He's an oatmeal and salad fiend—not together—and when he talks about building the perfect salad in the dinner chapter (see Chapter 8), I can almost guarantee that you'll be salivating.

**Jeremy Powers:** Powers is arguably the top guy in U.S. cyclocross—and one of the first to be able to race cyclocross for a living in the United States. He lives in western Massachusetts (when he's home), and as a pro cyclist, he's constantly focused on the perfect, dialed-in nutrition. His diet excludes nearly all processed foods and has a heavy emphasis on fruits and vegetables. It doesn't exclude anything whole.

**Mo Bruno Roy:** Bruno Roy is a recently retired pro cyclocrosser, and her specific approach to eating also encompasses the general philosophy of overall healthy, simple, whole foods. A vegan for the past 5 years and a vegetarian long before that, Bruno Roy isn't the kind of vegan who opts for soy-based chicken sandwiches. Instead, she focuses on a diet high in fruits and vegetables. She prefers to spend her money on good organic produce (and the occasional pricey juice) and uses nuts and beans as her main sources of protein. Despite the fact that her diet avoids all animal products, her diet closely resembles that of Powers or King. Bruno Roy is a two-time Singlespeed National Champion in cyclocross, she's raced at the World Championships for years, and she won the Singlespeed Cyclocross World Championships in 2014.

**Tayler Wiles:** Pro road racer Wiles loves food so much that her blog is completely packed with recipes ranging from fancy dinners to sweet breads that she eats as her own in-ride food. She may be a self-described cookie monster, but the cookies are all home-baked and made with the best-quality ingredients. Wiles is a roadie who started as a soccer player and a runner before discovering a natural aptitude for the bike. It was through pro bike racing that she met her girlfriend, a fellow pro racer who's gluten-free due to celiac disease. Because of this, Wiles eats a primarily gluten-free diet, but she's not a big fan of the gluten-free product craze. She prefers natural foods and simple recipes to premade gluten-free pizza crust, any day of the week.

Don't forget, these are racers putting in big hours on a weekly basis, so some of their meals can be a bit more calorically dense than someone who rides for 8 hours per week. As Guest will say over and over, nutrition is a highly individualized thing, and "personal case studies can't be used in place of objective science." The pros all have fantastic advice; just remember that what works for one pro racer may not work for you.

Onward!

# FUEL YOUR RIDE

# PART ONE

---

# THE BIG STUFF

Before we can start talking about the optimal breakfast, lunch, dinner, or ride food, it's important to understand exactly what goes into these three meals, and where we're getting our fuel. I'm the first person to admit that, for years, I had no idea what a fat, protein, or carbohydrate really was. I only knew what each was in the most general sense. I didn't know how they worked together or separately and, as such, I was incredibly susceptible to fancy-sounding diets that promised to work wonders if I just started eating A and X at Y and Z times, gave up B altogether, and only ate C in between the hours of 12:00 midnight and 1:00 a.m.

That's why it's so important to learn about what each one is: So the next time someone tells you about the latest elimination diet that cuts out a whole nutrient group, you know exactly what you'll be missing out on. A cyclist can't live on carbs alone, but he also can't live on protein or fat alone, either.

We aren't all the same, and this book will repeat over and over that you have to experiment to find out what works best for you. Our genes react differently to different foods, and that genetic influence can really impact your ideal breakdown of protein, carbohydrates, and fat. "The future is going to be considering your unique DNA to decide what the best type of training is for you, what the best way to lose weight is, and what diet is best for you," explains Nanci Guest, MSc, RD, CSCS.

This book lays the groundwork for what a healthy diet should look like, and as you get closer and closer to your cycling goals and your ideal weight by focusing on the principles outlined here, you can start to play around by slowly shifting and adding a bit more protein, or adjusting the carbohydrate ratios in your diet to see how your body reacts. It's a process, but look at your nutrition and training as a science experiment. Here, we're presenting the hypothesis and the experiment, but it's up to you to take the results and learn from them, tweak the experiment, and find the perfect solution for you.

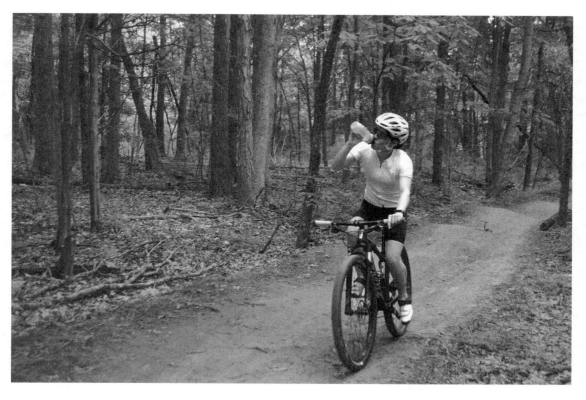

You have to be willing to experiment to get your fueling down to a science. Maybe you need a hydration pack on your mountain bike, or maybe a bottle is right for you.

# CHAPTER ONE

# WHY DOES IT MATTER?

Nutrition doesn't start on the bike. Every single person—racers, nutritionists, and coaches—I talked to said this over and over, so it's worth repeating. On your race day, or that epic endurance ride you have marked on your calendar, your breakfast and ride fuel are only a small part of the equation. How you've been eating for the past few months plays a huge role, not just in body composition, but in how you digest, how you use energy, and how you perform. You wouldn't start training the morning of a race, would you? So why should your nutrition start then?

The first thing we want to focus on is where we are now. Without knowing how well (or poorly) you're eating, it's hard to know what to tweak to fix your diet. And when it comes to macronutrient breakdown, most people are surprised by what the breakdown actually looks like for their daily diets. Hint: Carbohydrates and fat sneak in more often than you

think, whether you cook a lot at home or eat at restaurants for every meal.

What is a macronutrient? Macronutrients make up our food, and the big three are fat, protein, and carbohydrates. They work together to keep our bodies running. *Carbohydrates* fill up glycogen stores so we have energy to function and to ride; *fat* provides energy as well and helps to protect our cells and dissolve certain vitamins, while *protein* builds and repairs muscle—not just bodybuilder muscle, cyclist muscle, too.

In the next three chapters, we're breaking down these three into bite-size pieces (pun emphatically intended) so you know just how much of each to eat, the best time to eat each one, and the best options in each. Macronutrients aren't created equal; there are good and bad fats, proteins, and carbohydrates. Let's get started so we can cut out the bad and begin focusing on the good.

## YOUR BEST BIKE BODY

This is the big question for cyclists. What the heck is a bike body anyway? Is it one where your quads are so huge that you need specially tailored jeans to fit over your bulging muscles, or is it one so slender that even the tightest of skinny jeans are sagging off of your thin frame? Unfortunately, there's no one right answer, and like much of nutrition, it's all about the individual, as Smart Athlete coach (and slim but reasonably muscular elite racer) Peter Glassford explains.

"It's a complicated question—it depends on the sport you want to participate in," he admits. "There are a bunch of different sports within cycling, from ultra-endurance road cycling to multiday stage events to a track cycling event that may only last a couple of minutes. So there is a wide range of body types in cycling, not just skinny arms and huge legs."

Thank goodness.

But there are a few generalities that he shares.

**Road Cycling:** A road cyclist will typically be leaner, with not much muscle, low body fat, and much less upper body strength. Keeping weight low is even more important when you're doing more hilly rides and races versus flatter criterium races—to be successful, you have to watch out and keep weight low and muscle to a minimum. Not that strength training or consuming protein is bad, but you don't want to overconsume protein or do activities that tend to bulk up the upper body.

**Mountain Biking:** For mountain biking, on the other hand, you need a bit more muscle and upper body strength to navigate the varied terrain. It is common to see a mountain biker with a little more weight than your average road cyclist.

**Track Cycling:** This one is pretty variable, but generally, you'll see a more muscular sprinter body, similar to a running sprinter. It's very much power based, so having more muscle in the legs is key. They tend

Look at this first task the same way you would look at creating a household budget: You can't make a reasonable budget if you don't have a clue where the money is going right now, can you? A food diary is a great place to start. Even if you're not trying to lose weight and are simply trying to appropriately fuel your workouts, keeping a food diary for a few days to make sure you're getting enough calories, or to see if you are consuming too many (and to see what your nutritional macronutrient makeup is), is an easy, cheap, and noncommittal way to to be a bit bigger, but still pretty lean.

Glassford adds that when it comes to women, while the body types are similar to those we just described, there's a higher tendency toward outliers in the field. Just look at a women's professional field, and you'll see what he means. Tall, short, muscular, slender—there are so many different body types that can fit the winning bill for professional women's cycling. Even among the women interviewed for this book, there are huge discrepancies. "You see a much wider variation than you do in the men in terms of body types," Glassford says, and he's completely right.

But that just leads to the next point. Ride and eat right and your ideal cycling body type will find you. You can't change your DNA, but you can make your body most effective by—no surprise here—doing what you want it to do, and gradually letting it change. You wouldn't lift Olympic weights to get ready for a marathon, so why would you push heavy gears on the track if you're hoping to be a climbing specialist on the road?

"The sport takes care of it—whatever discipline you do the most of is how your body will start to develop," Glassford explains. "But you are limited a bit by your frame. That shouldn't discourage anyone though— there are outliers all the time. You see people make what they're born with work well—a smaller, more muscular racer may be great at cyclocross, where being a little more built muscularly can help with lifting the bike over the barriers, running with the bike, and staying steady on the bike through the mud. There's always a discipline for you . . . or a technique that lets you compete in the discipline that you want to be in."

So before you throw this book out because you're afraid you'll never make it as a pro roadie because you pack on muscle like a linebacker heading into training camp, don't panic. There's still hope.

get a snapshot of where your diet is. You can use a notebook, a spreadsheet, or one of the countless free fitness apps available on your smartphone. Pro cyclocrosser Jeremy Powers swears by MyFitnessPal, but choose whatever one you will actually use.

"You don't just know all of this nutrition stuff," Powers says when he talks about why he records what he eats and why he cares about the nutritional makeup of his food. "You have to be in a place where you make time to learn and to cook. I don't think any rider just immediately starts doing this. But I knew, for me, it was something I needed to do to get to the next level and keep my body healthy. And as I get older, I need to be on top of that."

Once you've recorded a few days of normal eating, you should be able to see patterns emerge. Maybe you have a huge breakfast, but don't go for a ride until midafternoon. Or, are you a late-night snacker because you train later in the day but eat a small dinner? Are you eating way more calories than you thought, or far less? Are you drinking enough water, or too much coffee? We make food choices that may not be the smartest (like that midday muffin 30 minutes before lunch) when we're not thinking about what we're doing, and having a written log is a great way of both taking note of those tendencies and working to curtail them.

The good news: Keeping a log isn't something you need to do forever. Think of it as an occasional exercise in mindfulness. "You do it, and then you take a step back the following season and say, 'Okay, that was good.' You begin to recognize where your nutrients are coming from," says retired pro road racer Ted King. "I think cyclists, in general, have their ears to the ground, so to speak, and understand nutrition. I love my time in the kitchen. I love paying attention to food, so, inherently, I look at a pile of cashews and now I just know roughly how much fat, protein, and carbs are in it. It might sound nerdy, but at this point, it's second nature. So, I inherently understand it, and I don't really need to nerd out on that stuff anymore."

As King points out, keeping a food diary can create long-term results. Even if you only keep it for a few days, observing serving sizes in relation to the portion size you are eating will give you a better sense of how many calories you are actually eating.

Pro cyclocrosser Katie Compton is a fan of keeping a food diary, and not just for counting calories. She's experienced some health and allergy issues over the years, and having a comprehensive log of what she ate and when she ate it has helped her adjust her diet into something that makes her feel good—something she needs when racing weekly through the fall and winter.

"I've been keeping a food diary for a few years now," she says. "It helps me keep track of when I'm feeling shitty and what I ate. Sometimes, you forget, especially when traveling and racing. You try to think back, but you can't remember everything that you had, so it's nice to have the diary to look back on." Laughing at herself, she admits, "but keeping it is annoying as hell, and I hate it."

Now that you know roughly how much food you're eating each day, it's time to see if that's too much, too little, or just about right. "When working with an athlete, I like to start with determining their overall calorie needs," explains Alexa McDonald, RD, CDN. "Those needs are often elevated in cyclists and other endurance athletes because of the intensity and duration of the sport. I break down their caloric needs into three different meals and two or three snacks per day, with taking into consideration and making some exceptions based on timing, duration, and frequency of their training."

To do this, you'll begin by calculating your basal metabolic rate (BMR)—a rough estimate of what you burn in a day before any activity. It's pretty simple, actually: For women, your BMR is your weight in pounds multiplied by 9.9; for men, weight is multiplied by 10.8. That's about how many calories you need in a day to just exist.

Now, here's where you can do one of two things. For an easy calculation to take exercise into account, multiply your BMR by 1.5, and if you consider yourself very active (training hard on a daily basis), multiply it by 1.7. If you'd prefer a more accurate count, simply multiply your BMR by 1.2 (the measurement for someone who's inactive) if you work a desk job and rarely are active except for training, or by 1.3 if you're fairly mobile even outside of training. Then, calculate how much you burn on the bike. This can be done using one of the many online calorie calculators available. (*Bicycling* magazine has a great calculator on their website.[1]) Or use your heart rate monitor or power meter to give you the most accurate reading. Got a number? Add it to that original BMR calculation, and voilà! The number of calories you burn in a given day.

If you're trying to maintain weight, make sure you stay fairly close to that number. If you're trying to gain weight, go a bit higher, and if you're trying to lose weight, go a bit lower—but more on that later.

First, let's get into the nitty-gritty science of what you're putting in your body and why you're doing it. We're going to break down the three major macronutrients: protein, fat, and carbohydrates. Each one of them is important—especially for cyclists—and each has been demonized in the past few decades for one reason or another. In the 1980s, fat took the blame for the growing obesity epidemic in America, so we introduced a lot of low- and no-fat foods to combat that. But to make the foods still taste good, since fat is admittedly delicious, we crammed those chemically engineered monstrosities with sugar.

When the obesity epidemic seemed to take off even more in the early 2000s, we decided to blame carbohydrates and sugar. Now, it seems like no one can agree on which is the greatest evil ... but luckily, as a cyclist in training, there simply isn't one evil of the three macronutrients. Why are all three important, and why do we need them? It all comes down to energy.

When we talk about burning energy during exercise, we're not just making a killer metaphor. We're talking about splitting the bond in ATP (adenosine triphosphate, for those science geeks) molecules, which then releases energy as it loses one of its phosphate groups and becomes

ADP (adenosine diphosphate). Don't worry—we won't nerd out too much here, but it is important to understand the basics of what energy really is and why we need it.

In cycling, at some point or another, every rider has experienced bonking—that feeling of hitting a wall, where your legs suddenly become too heavy to pedal, your mood plummets, and you just need a ride to be over. That's not a psychological issue (though, admittedly, sometimes it's more mental than physical, especially when the weather is bad or the ride isn't going according to plan). Bonking means you're out of energy stores, and your body is going into crisis mode. We want to avoid running out of energy at all costs, but at the same time, we want to avoid overfeeding, which can sadly make a ride lead to a net caloric gain versus a loss. You don't want all that hard work to be for nothing, do you?

"You hear a lot about the 80:20 rule, where you can eat 80 percent well and 20 percent indulgent, and if you're just the average person who does the basic requirement of trying to get out for 30 minutes most days of the week, and you don't care if you're carrying an extra 10 pounds, that's fine," Nanci Guest, MSc, RD, CSCS, explains. "You can get by being a bit more relaxed. But for optimal health, people should really be more so following a 90:10 rule, and the 10 percent is really about psychology more than anything else. You don't want to be so disciplined you're making sacrifices that make you unhappy."

"Then there are the people who want to lean out, who want that six-pack, who want to see improvements in their performance, and they're more 95:5," she adds. "And if you're at the highest level, if you want to get to that goal the fastest and most efficient way, you have to be disciplined." When Guest consults with athletes who are aiming for the Olympics, she often tells them "I'm sorry, but you need to be at the 100:0 ratio. You can always be assured that someone is working a little harder and eating a little better than you, and that will be the difference between gold and silver. A gold-medal athlete sacrifices everything. You can control your level of discipline and level of commitment."

So it's up to you, really. How important is that cupcake?

## YOUR DIET TYPE

Fad diets are in. That's undeniable. But it's rare to see a pro cyclist who follows a specific diet. If they do follow one, as in the case of vegan retired pro cyclocrosser Mo Bruno Roy, the description of her diet sounds eerily similar to that of omnivorous Powers, who does not follow a specific diet.

Powers explains his diet saying, "The only thing that I put in my body is nutrient-dense foods. So no cereal or things that have sugar calories. Generally, I don't eat anything unless it has a lot of color in it and came from the earth or an animal. There are a lot of processed foods that I don't eat anymore."

Bruno Roy's philosophy? Eat as much as possible in its natural state.

What every pro has in common is a disdain for highly-processed foods (except in competition situations, but more on that later). And while some opt to leave gluten out of their diets and others elect to stay animal product–free, even their meals are similar in description: lots of vegetables as a base, followed by a small amount of simple carbohydrate, and a moderate amount of protein—animal or otherwise. Sound simple? That's because it is.

"I don't really have a specific 'thing,'" pro road racer Tayler Wiles says, sounding confused that I even asked about a nutritional philosophy. She continues, "My partner, Olivia, is gluten-free, so we mostly are gluten-free, but I'll eat it during the season, because at races, it's really hard to be picky and choosy about what you eat. So I'll eat a little of everything so I'm not restricted. We try to eat real foods, though—nothing processed, and everything in moderation. I don't do any no fat or no carbs, just a well-balanced diet of whole foods."

There's that real-foods, nothing-processed thing again. If it sounds like a trend, or a constant refrain, that's because it is.

Even if you subscribe to one of these diets, like Paleo, there's still plenty to be gained by reading this book and thinking about modify-

ing that elimination diet to best fuel your riding. "Most approaches can work for most people, if you think about your overall health and a balance of nutrients," Guest says. But on the other hand, "if you're on a diet where you have to add Metamucil to each meal to get fiber, if you have to take a bunch of vitamins because it's not coming from your food—that's not health, that's not balance, and that's not the right approach. Anything that's too extreme will eventually be harmful in some way to your health or performance."

For example, Guest explains, "I see so many vegetarians and vegans eating boxed cereals and chips. Taking meat out of your diet doesn't automatically make your diet healthy."

Instead, opt for a healthy vegan diet like Bruno Roy's, one that's based on making sure most of her food comes from clean, natural sources and balances the macronutrients that she needs. "When you go to the grocery store— if you can afford to go to Whole Foods or a farmers' market or a local co-op or something, great—just start looking at the food," she suggests. "Look at the food in as close to its natural state as possible. Then, when you pick up something that's packaged, just realize how many steps away it is from the thing that grew out of the ground. You may still be fine with it and buy it, but you'll have a better awareness of the distance it's gone from its natural state."

Sound too difficult to switch over to all-healthy all the time? "Once a week," Bruno Roy

*(continues on page 15)*

# CAN I GO VEGAN?

Vegan retired pro cyclocrosser Mo Bruno Roy is just one individual in the growing population of vegan athletes who are performing at the pro level. She's been a vegan for 5 years and, as both a cyclist and a yoga instructor, she's completely in tune with her body's needs.

Here, she shares her story and highlights the importance of a clean vegan diet versus one full of meat substitutes and highly processed foods.

"I've been vegan for 5 years, but I was vegetarian for 10 years before that," she explains. "I grew up on a farm where we raised our own food—chickens, turkeys, that kind of stuff. Then, my twin sister and I went to college, and it was the first time we had really eaten processed food, which is surprising because every kid eats candy and junk food once in a while, but we never did for regular meals until then. And we both got really sick, had terrible digestive issues, and things like that. Luckily, we were living in a suite with a little kitchenette, so our parents ended up giving us a bunch of food like rice and frozen vegetables from home, and we just ate that. Because I was having such a hard time digesting these processed foods I hadn't eaten before, like meat that wasn't from a farm, within a year, I stopped eating meat, in general. So it was easy for

me to be vegetarian. Once I left my parents' house, I just didn't eat it anymore."

For Bruno Roy, at first, it was less about eating no animal products as opposed to knowing from where those products came. "I always knew where my food came from, so it was easy for me to decide that if I didn't know where it came from, I wasn't going to eat it. I learned a lot about different farming practices, and it was easy for me to see that veganism was right for me. For me, it was easy—I never even liked eggs! We grew up with these awesome hens who gave us eggs, but I wasn't into eggs, and I never really cared for cheese or milk. I can't think of much that I miss, so it was a pretty easy transition for me."

"When I started, there were no restaurants that were vegan in Boston—it's more of a sports town with tons of sports teams. Fish is big, so there weren't a lot of options for me to eat out. But I love cooking at home anyway, so it's not a big deal," she explains.

Unfortunately for many of us, we didn't grow up on a farm or avoiding some of the junk food that Bruno Roy did, so we have a bit more of a taste for it. "I think, in general, my eating habits were very clean growing up," she remembers. "Everything has a label now, slow food or macrobiotic or whatever, but that's what I just grew up with: real food.

Even labeling something vegan or vegetarian doesn't seem to have such a direct health impact anymore—I never replaced things. For me, it was just leaving things out and making sure my meals were balanced, not adding in a bunch of fake stuff."

"I've always done clean eating," she says, and that's impacted her recovery and immunity her entire life. "I've always been the person who gets only one head cold a year. I've been really lucky."

If you're considering going vegan, and you don't already have basic cooking skills, now is the time to learn them. "If you don't cook, it's really hard, especially to eat ethically and be a vegan. If you don't cook— some people hate cooking and I find that amazing because I love it—you need alternatives, and that usually involves frozen stuff with a lot of preservatives and sodium, and you lose the quality of the foods."

It's possible to balance the principles outlined in this book with eschewing animal products, but that doesn't mean going for the vegan chicken wings. It's more about opting for healthy substitutes such as chickpeas instead of a steak. Bruno Roy's biggest tip, whether you are planning on becoming a vegan or already are one, is to be on top of current research and really know what your diet is about. "It's great to read current research," she says, "and to be in charge and understand the unconventional or conventional diet that you choose."

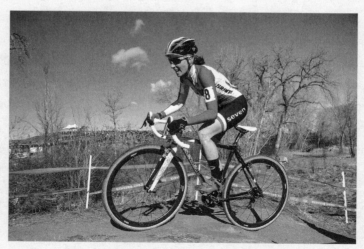

Mo Bruno Roy is committed to being vegan, and she does it in a way that fuels her rides perfectly and leaves her feeling great.

# ANTIOXIDANTS—THE PROS AND CONS

An antioxidant actually has a real purpose, in addition to being that buzzword you hear tossed around when superfoods are being listed (blueberries! goji berries! raspberries! white cherries!—the more obscure the food is, the more likely it is to make it into a top-10 foods list these days). The question that's been steadily becoming more and more prevalent in the nutrition community is: Do antioxidants really matter?

"Antioxidants are molecules that counter free radicals, which are free hydrogen molecules," explains nutritionist Jordan Dubé, MS. "Antioxidants are missing a hydrogen, so they accept those free radicals to form a larger molecule."

So, antioxidants bind free radicals, but why do we have free radicals in the first place? This is where the role of antioxidants in an athlete's diet—at least, in large doses—gets dicey. Recent studies are showing that direct supplementation with antioxidants during training is interfering with training-induced adaptations caused by free radicals. Because we actually need a low level of free radicals in order to stimulate change in our muscles, using antioxidants to bind the free radicals can actually do as much harm as it can good.

Does this mean we should give up blueberries altogether? Of course not. But ingesting huge doses of foods that are jammed with antioxidants isn't the best plan when you're right in the middle of trying to increase your VO$_2$ max.

Of course, what you've heard about antioxidants is likely not even truly about antioxidants, since it's become such a blanket term. "*Antioxidant* is an overused term," explains Nanci Guest, MSc, RD, CSCS. "Even though they're important to our health and we get them from foods, nutrition researchers are backing away from the claims made about them boosting brainpower or fighting cancer. Now, they're looking at phytochemicals from fruits and plants and seeing what else they do in the body, like acting as anti-inflammatories. You shouldn't look at labels and assume you need things high in antioxidants anymore. Superfoods with antioxidants don't really fly in nutritional physiology circles anymore."

The moral of the story is simple: Just because that bottle of juice says it's full of antioxidants and costs $10, that doesn't mean it's a superfood. It won't do anything for your training session that a homemade fruit smoothie won't do.

suggests, "try to eat only things in their natural states. I always recommend starting with once a week, or even one meal per week."

Once you do start switching to a more natural diet, though, beware. Just because it's natural doesn't mean that the calories don't count. "People often get confused about healthy foods versus low-calorie foods," says Guest. "First of all, just because a food is labeled low calorie doesn't mean it's nutritious or contributing anything valuable toward your performance goals and/or health, especially if it's a highly-processed version of something, like nonfat low-sugar yogurt. On the other hand, there are plenty of healthy foods that are packed with calories, like avocados or nuts and seeds. Even bananas have a lot of calories for what they are. So just because something is natural doesn't mean you should just eat a ton of it. It will still have calories. Whatever you eat, healthy or not, will have calories."

## IT'S ALL ABOUT TIMING

Unfortunately, this book isn't going to be able to give you a one-size-fits-all diet plan. No one can. However, this book does have plenty of information about how much of each macronutrient you need to eat at certain times and why it's important. Even ratios of carbohydrates to protein to fat are too general and inaccurate to include. A ratio won't do you much good if you're eating all protein while on the bike,

a fatty recovery meal, and then a big bowl of carbohydrate-filled pasta for dinner. It all comes down to timing, and eating the right amounts at those right times.

"Matching nutrition to training is really important to maximize fuel and recovery to maximize the benefits of a training session or for leaning out," Guest says. You can't talk about sports nutrition without discussing nutrient timing. Otherwise, you could end up eating the same 1,000-calorie breakfast as pro road racer Janel Holcomb, only to sit at the office the rest of the day while Holcomb, who fueled specifically for her ride, is out on an endurance ride for the better part of the day.

Nutrient timing doesn't just mean how you schedule your day. As cyclists, we tend to take more time off in the winter, especially those of us who live in climates where riding outside isn't possible or pleasant year-round. No one likes working out on an indoor trainer. Your hours in the winter are likely less than your hours in the summer, as they should be to properly rest, recover, and get excited for the next season.

Since we ride less in the winter, our caloric needs are lower, so our diets need to shift. The winter is also a great chance for athletes to focus on building that lean body mass and dropping fat. "If you're periodizing your training, consider taking the winter for some quality gym time," Guest says. "Things like strength and power training are great, as well as some much-needed stretching sessions to undo the muscle tightness that you accumulated over the season.

"You don't train the same way all year, so you shouldn't eat the same all year," she says. And for those of you who think the winter off-season means a chance to really let loose, think again. Those decisions will likely come back to bite you in the (slightly doughy) butt come May and competition time. "You shouldn't start addressing nutrition just before a competition. What have you been doing the rest of the year? Anything you do now will affect you in 6 months, and at the cellular level, what you're doing to take care of yourself now is going to result in better performance in 3 months, in 6 months, in a year."

So look at it as two types of nutrition rather than one all-encompassing, slightly terrifying idea of nutrition as a whole. You have long-term nutrition and the minute day-to-day nutrition, or to put it slightly more scientifically, "We have chronic nutrition and acute nutrition," Guest explains. "So, today, if I don't get enough carbs or water, my training session is going to suffer. But today's training session won't be affected if I didn't have enough iron today or enough protein yesterday. There are some things that take a longer time to have an effect. That's why every day you want to think about doing the right thing, to build a good foundation at the cellular level, and provide that nutritional support to whatever your training goals are."

## CHAPTER TWO

# FAT

Before we tackle how to plan out a day's worth of eating, it's important to understand why we need certain macronutrients—fat, protein, and carbohydrates. And to kick it off, we'll start with the one with the most caloric density at 9 calories per gram: fat.

Fat is the easiest of the macronutrients to demonize—the name says it all, right?

Absolutely not.

In fact, more and more people are beginning to subscribe to high-fat diets, and not just crazed diet fanatics: There are some well-known endurance athletes who swear by it. While that approach may work for some, it's certainly not for everyone, and there are major pitfalls to having an extremely low-carb diet. That said, one thing that we've learned is that fat is essential to a healthy diet, especially for athletes, since it's used to manufacture tissues and hormones, insulate our bodies, and protect our organs and cells.

A fat, at its most basic, is a compound made up of a chain of fatty acids. It provides energy as well as protection to our cells. Additionally, we need fat to break down certain fat-soluble vitamins like vitamins A, D, and E, which our bodies can't break down with water alone.

Fats have a bad rap for a reason, so don't assume that just because some people are proponents of high-fat diets that any style of oil, lard, or butter is good for you. Some fats are healthier than others, and some should be avoided or at least used in extreme moderation. The simple rule of thumb is that saturated fats are often linked to problems like heart disease, while poly- and monounsaturated fats are associated with good fats.

And then there is the worst offender when it comes to unhealthy fats: Fast food often contains trans fat, which is a fat that has gone through a hydrogenation process to give it a longer shelf life. You can, for the most part, avoid trans fat by avoiding greasy fried food and any ultra-processed snack foods made with partially hydrogenated oils. (You should be avoiding these anyway!)

Fat is a cornerstone in any successful, healthy diet. For cyclists, we spend much of our time munching on simple carbs on the bike, so it stands to reason that balancing out that sugary overload with healthy fats during the rest of our day is important to a balanced, clean diet.

"Eating low fat and high carbohydrate is the worst advice I've gotten," says pro cyclo-crosser Katie Compton, who's been winning Nationals for more than a decade. She has her nutrition down to a science, and she adds that putting fat back into her diet was a game-changer. "As long as you're picking healthy fat sources like coconut oil or grass-fed butter or avocados, you're fine. Eating fat keeps you less hungry and your body burns more efficiently. You don't want to eat a hamburger and fries every day to increase your fat intake, but adding in healthy fats is important."

## WHAT KIND OF FAT DO I NEED?

As I've already mentioned, some fats are better than others. That said, most foods containing fats harbor several different types of fats, so even when you think you're getting all good fat, you're likely getting a dose of a less-than-amazing one at the same time. "We don't have pure specific fats," explains Nanci Guest, MSc, RD, CSCS. "We just label based on which is the predominant fat in the mixture."

The good news is that it's the mixture of fats that you need. "It's good to get a variety," Guest adds. "People can't just eat 20 almonds a day and call it good; you're missing out on other important nutrients. You have to change it up, and the more variety you get, the wider profile of nutrients you're getting."

Before you go out and get that burger and fries thinking it'll provide that good fat though, let's break it down a bit more.

## Omega-3s and Omega-6s

"The fats that you need should take priority in your diet," Guest says. "You want to choose fats that are essential: omega-3s and omega-6s. They're essential because we can't make them," she explains.

These are the fats—especially if your goal is to build or maintain your weight—that you want to add in. "Add fat if you need to meet a calorie quota," says Guest, "and to improve the nutrient density of that quota, fats are essential."

It all comes down to not wasting those precious calories on bad fats like saturated or trans fats. "If I have 2,000 calories to work with, I don't want to spend 15 percent of that on saturated fats because then I'm wasting those calories on something that isn't adding any nutritional benefits," Guest explains. "That's what ends the argument for me: There's nothing in saturated fat that we need to give us a health benefit we can't get any-where else. If you enjoy it because it tastes good, that's your call. But there's no good rea-son, other than psychological, to integrate saturated fats instead of omegas into your diet plan. Don't believe the headlines that satu-rated fat isn't bad for you and won't hurt you—it's still calories that aren't helping your health. There's nothing in it that's growing your muscles."

Where do you get omega-3s? They're a little harder to find than saturated fats, or even omega-6s. "Omega-3s aren't in a lot of things. They're probably the most difficult one to get, so people should look at sources like flaxseeds and fish," says Guest.

We've learned a lot about the need for omega-3s in recent years, and it's no longer the standard to use the sources we once did. "It was thought that we needed fish oil, and we were saying that you couldn't get docosa-hexaenoic acid (DHA), alpha-linolenic acid (ALA), or omega-3s from plant sources," says Guest. "But now, we're only seeing that veg-ans are 20 percent lower in DHA. So it seems that people can get everything that they require from plant sources, though the most direct source is certainly fish and fish oil."

Omega-6s, on the other hand, can be found in most processed foods. "We get plenty of them," Guest says. "So unless you stick to a low-fat diet or eat no processed foods, you don't

have to worry about supplementing at all. Peo-ple should also focus on making their omega-3 to omega-6 ratio as close to 1:1 as possible, but the average American diet is closer to 1:10, with an overdose of omega-6."

## Ain't Nothing like the Real Thing

You may be shocked to realize that coconut oil, olive oil, walnut oil . . . any oil, really, is pro-cessed. Actually, that shouldn't be a huge sur-prise. That's common sense. But so many lists of superfoods have led us to believe that olive oil and coconut oil are going to change our lives. So it's easy to mistake them for a diet sta-ple. But what about their natural state? You know, actually eating those coconuts, olives, and walnuts.

"The question always is, how can I get the most nutritional bang for my buck?" says Guest. "So, for example, if I eat olive oil, I'm missing out on some of the good stuff that's in olives. Or if I'm getting the processed form of flaxseed in oil, I'm missing out on a lot of the antioxidants and protein and a lot of things in the flaxseed that provide health benefits and are lost when we just consume the oil."

She continues, "There's something to be said about getting fats in their natural state. If we can go back to fats in their natural state, that's a way to get them in the most nutritious form along with other benefits. I think going back to the source is a great shift for most people."

And admittedly, we're still going to use these oils for cooking, baking, and dressings for salads. We aren't monsters. But maybe consider keeping the oil consumption lower and trying to get those fats from a more natural source. It'll be more filling to eat a cup of olives (yum!) than to use a tablespoon of olive oil. "I know no one can eat a cup of olives every day, but it's a good exercise to try to incorporate more of the natural form," Guest adds, "especially when it comes from nuts or seeds or avocados. If you can go back to the source, you get so much more nutrition." And if you're using avocado oil instead of enjoying avocados, you might be in need of the awesome guacamole recipe that is featured in this chapter. "I try to shift people away from eating many oils and try to shift them into getting their fats from something that also has other nutrients so you can get more health benefits," Guest concludes.

## THE NO-FLY ZONE: BAD FATS
### Saturated Fats

Saturated fats have a bad rap, and it's for a good reason. They're the ones found in fatty meats, cheese, and whole milk. They tend to be solid at room temperature. (That bacon grease you left sitting in the pan in the morning? Yeah, that's saturated fat.) And while the bad news is that there's nothing good about

them, the good news is that we don't actually need them at all.

"The body can make saturated fats," Guest explains, "and so, we can exist on a diet of zero saturated fats. It's not an essential fat, so if you're going to look at the ones that are important to a diet, this isn't one of them."

If you're looking to cut calories, this is a smart place to start. Aim for lean meats and nonfat dairy products—but that said, a little flavor goes a long way, so if you're craving that burger, go for it—just don't make it a habit.

"There's a lot of literature about how saturated fats can raise your bad LDL cholesterol," Guest explains. "There's no argument there, the argument is whether that bad cholesterol actually raises your risk of a heart attack. But new research is showing that while high LDL cholesterol is a high risk factor for a heart attack or heart disease, not everyone who has a heart attack or heart disease actually has high LDL cholesterol. We can agree that there is a risk, though."

Saturated fats, especially if you're looking to lean out, are not important to your diet, so look where you can cut them out. Do you really need that bacon with your morning eggs? "Most people are looking to get lean or to stay lean—to keep lean muscle mass and drop body fat," adds Guest. "So you need to make sure that your nutrition is matching that goal. If you have 200 calories a day coming from

# THE UNDEMONIZATION OF FAT [AND CARBS]

Today, we no longer view fat as the ultimate evil and, instead, we blame carbohydrates as the new cause of all obesity and disease. And while there are certainly problems with both carbs and fats, it's time for the demonization of any one macronutrient to stop.

"In the eighties, the American Heart Association came out with all this information about fat and how it was going to kill you: giving you cancer and heart disease, making you sick, making you fat," explains nutritionist Jordan Dubé, MS.

The reaction to this public outcry, however, was even worse than the problem. "Then, in response, we got all of these processed, low-fat foods," she explains. Low- and no-fat food options became popular as the general public bought into diet-friendly alternatives to their favorite guilty pleasures—think SnackWell's cookies. But as with all quick fixes, there were serious consequences. "Americans basically removed fat from their diets and replaced it with tons and tons of processed carbs and added sugars to every single thing that they ate," says Dubé. "There's pretty strong evidence that eating like this made everyone even sicker, and we need fat in our diets."

You'd think after 30 years, we would have learned to find moderation in all things, but it's not so easy, especially for athletic people. "It's still ingrained in athletes' minds, who are taught that as active people, we need higher carbohydrate rations than the average person," Dubé says. "But the problem with that is that the average person eats far too many carbohydrates. So if you're eating the average diet plus more carbs, you're in trouble. You're never going to drop that extra weight."

Yes, athletes need carbs but probably not as many as you may think. More important, they need to eat the right carbs at the right times.

Moral of the story? Stop demonizing any single macronutrient and, instead, eat all three in moderation and at the appropriate time.

# Killer Good Guac

Avocados: Almost every pro lists avocados as one of their favorite foods, and for good reason. In addition to being delicious, avocados are an excellent source of healthy fats. In fact, a recent study showed that including an avocado as a daily part of a moderate-fat diet can lower cholesterol. Avocados are a nutrient-dense source of monounsaturated fatty acids and, therefore, can actually lower low-density lipoprotein (LDL) cholesterol when replacing saturated fats in a person's diet.

To add healthy fats, fiber, potassium, and vitamins C, K, and B$_6$ (and plenty more) into your diet, try topping your lunch or dinner with guacamole. It's not just for dipping tortilla chips: It's a great salad topper if you're craving a creamy dressing; it livens up rice and beans; and it's delicious with sweet potato fries. As an added bonus, this recipe sneaks in a ton of veggies, so the fat and calorie content are lower than traditional guacamole. Use more onions and tomatoes if you are trying to keep your calories per serving lower.

- 2 ripe avocados (they should be nice and malleable when you squeeze them, but not mushy)
- 2 tablespoons fresh lime juice (from about 1 lime)
- 1–2 tomatoes, finely chopped
- ½–1 red onion, finely chopped
- Sea salt, to taste
- Handful of cilantro, roughly chopped

Peel and pit the avocados. Mash them in a bowl. Add the lime juice, tomatoes, onion, salt, and cilantro and toss together.

Sounds simple, right? It will make you a hero at parties, family dinners, or even to yourself when you're eating alone after a long day.

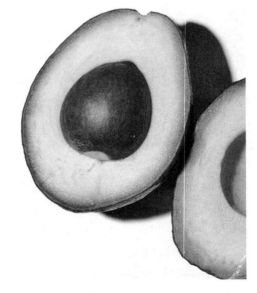

Make guacamole your go-to for an easy snack that's full of healthy fats, tastes great, and will be the hit of the party!

saturated fat, that's 200 calories that can be allocated somewhere else that will be better, whether it's more carbs on the bike or more protein to build lean muscle or even just healthier fats."

## Trans Fats

Now we're talking the worst of the worst. There are actually laws in place banning this fat. And in America, home of the Big Mac, Gulp, and a whole bunch of other excessively named food items, it must be pretty darn bad when Republicans and Democrats can come together and agree that one thing isn't healthy—that it's bad enough to ban. "When it comes to bad fats, the top bad fat is trans fat,"

### SNEAKING HEALTHY FATS INTO YOUR DIET

Alexa McDonald, RD, CDN, lists a few great options to inject healthy fats in your diet:

- 3-ounce portion of fatty fish, like salmon, mackerel, cod, rainbow trout, albacore tuna, or halibut (about 2 servings per week)

- 2 tablespoons natural peanut butter

- ¼ cup mixed nuts (for example, almonds, walnuts, and pistachios)

- ⅓ avocado

- 1 or 2 eggs

says Guest. "It's unhealthy for the heart and the immune system. It's a man-made fat that's been chemically altered, that the body doesn't accept, and that should be avoided. It's been banned in cities for use in restaurants. There are laws against it."

## HOW DO I EAT IT?

Fat is essential for any person, but for athletes, it is even more important. Since fat has 9 calories per gram, it offers more bang for your caloric buck, which can be hugely important if you're putting in long training hours. It also serves as extra fuel for your longer, endurance-paced rides.

"Due to the body's ability to store large amounts, fat becomes the major fuel for athletes about 2 hours into prolonged exercise," says Alexa McDonald, RD, CDN. "Athletes, like all individuals, should aim for 20 to 35 percent of their calories from fat. Most important, athletes want to focus on sources of healthy fats, such as avocados, fatty fish, olive oil, natural peanut butter, and nuts, with more than 10 percent of their calories coming from monounsaturated and polyunsaturated fats. While unhealthy fats, like saturated and trans fats, can still be consumed in moderation, they should be balanced out by choosing nutritious, high-quality sources that offer other benefits, such as red meats and low-fat cheeses. Keep in mind that saturated fats and trans fats should

(continues on page 26)

# THE PROBLEMS WITH A HIGH-FAT DIET

The latest in the fad diets seems to be the high-fat diets. You've likely seen the news stories about some athletes who are claiming to be "fat adapted," and in some—albeit very few—circumstances, that might work. But for a normal cyclist on a normal training schedule with an intention of going long and going fast, a high-fat diet isn't a great solution.

"You can do long, slow distance on a high-fat diet," Nanci Guest, MSc, RD, CSCS says. "But you'd have to be at a percentage below 70 percent of VO$_2$ max. In the studies that have been done, athletes were unable to sprint. When they exercised timed-to-exhaustion, they couldn't put out a big effort at the end of the exercise when exhausted. They simply couldn't push harder and sprint at the end of the effort."

This is because a body can't oxidize lipids fast enough with a higher power output, Guest explains. That means short efforts are largely carbohydrate-dependent. If you're running 100 miles, maybe a high-fat diet can get you through. But there simply isn't an upside to giving up carbs altogether.

"For performance, it's just not going to work," Guest explains. "In the off-season, there's the ability to use high fat to get leaner, but I think it's important to point out the importance of carb intake."

Alexa McDonald, RD, CDN, offers another take on why a high-fat diet may not be for you. "Unfortunately for the endurance athlete, fat alone cannot be used for energy during activity, and it requires the presence of carbohydrates to be effectively utilized," she says. "This is why continuing to fuel with carbohydrates during long workouts is especially necessary. Adequate glycogen stores [Glycogen is energy stored in the muscles and liver.] resulting from a high-carbohydrate diet have been shown to help increase endurance and intensity during performance."

It's exciting to think about some of the promises and claims made by proponents of the high-fat diet: The immediate weight loss promised is definitely intriguing, even for those of us who know better.

But doesn't it make more sense to fuel your ride the way you know will work for you versus taking a few months trying to force your body to adapt to something it doesn't really want to adapt to? High fat might be the answer for some people, but for you, the athlete, it's just not the best way to get fast.

And for women, female athlete physiology expert Stacy Sims, MSc, PhD, explains that a high-fat diet is even worse. "Things like intermittent fasting and high-fat diets aren't as good for women," she says. "They put a lot of stress on the body so we end up with higher levels of cortisol, and we end up with greater fatigue. And if you have a really high-fat diet to stay in ketosis [When in ketosis, the body starts producing ketones to create energy by breaking down fat instead of glycogen.], you have to have a lot of cortisol [the stress hormone] circulating, and you're in this high-stress state. The thing that cortisol does is it downplays muscle cell turnover and turns it down so you don't recover as well."

A stressed-out body and a poor recovery? That sounds . . . less than optimal. And sure, Dr. Sims admits that. "You might see results right away with a high-fat diet, but eventually, power will decline and you won't lean up as quickly because your cortisol levels will be up."

There are plenty of studies being done, but the results are all across the board. When it comes to a sustainable, long-term diet solution, it boils down to the fact that high fat just isn't for everyone. "Although some studies found longer time-to-exhaustion results during moderate-intensity workouts," McDonald notes, "most studies in this area found that while performance may be preserved with a high-fat diet, there was very little evidence of actual performance improvement."

"With this in mind, the effectiveness of this type of diet during training and performance may be best avoided or only indicated on an individual basis," McDonald

adds. "Workout intensity and timing, as well as performance goals and dietary preferences, should be taken into account by athletes as they determine the best training diet for them."

Just because you've read about high-fat diets or heard about some superathlete who swears by it, don't assume that it will work for you. The athletes who have experienced positive results from high-fat diets are generally long-distance athletes, as a rule, and often aren't working normal jobs in addition to their athletic careers.

And even if a high-fat diet did benefit your training, there hasn't been very much research on the long-term effects of switching to a high-fat diet.

Pro mountain biker Georgia Gould experienced the negative effects of a high-fat diet firsthand. "I tried a low-carb, high-fat diet once, and it was a very big fail for me," she recalls. "That was my one brush with that, and I realized it clearly wasn't working at all. So I went back to my old diet, which was no diet, just being smart and logical. You know, vegetables, good; processed food, bad." Any time that a diet ignores one of the three essential macronutrients, it's not a smart choice for your body, especially for athletes.

be kept to less than 10 percent and 1 percent of calories, respectively."

Fat is essential to our diets. That's simple enough. However, if you've ever tried to go for a ride after a big breakfast of bacon and eggs, you know it's not that simple. Since it takes a bit longer to digest than simple carbohydrates, it's not a great pre-ride food.

"Fat is something that should be eaten away from exercise," says Guest. "It doesn't matter as much when you eat it if you're not working out for a full 24 hours. Eating fiber and fat is fine if you're not planning on working out right away—then, you want to focus on replenishing glycogen stores, and you don't want fat to slow that down. So you don't want fat right before or right after exercise. Work around your training and just avoid it before and after."

A few grams of fat is not a problem, and plenty of in-ride bars even have a bit of fat in them, so don't panic. Just don't load up on anything high in fat for a few hours before a ride, and make sure that your post-ride carbs and protein are already in your system so that you're well on your way to recovery before adding a bunch of fat to slow down the process.

## YOUR FIVE TAKEAWAYS

1. Healthy fats are a cornerstone of any balanced diet.

2. Omega-3s and omega-6s are important in every diet, vegan or otherwise, and can be found in a wide variety of foods.

3. The more real-food fats you can eat instead of oils—especially from plant- and nut-based sources—the better.

4. You don't need saturated fats, and you should avoid trans fats. If you're trying to drop weight, remove these from your diet first.

5. Keep meals and snacks lighter on fats, especially those consumed pre-ride.

# CHAPTER THREE

# PROTEIN

P rotein isn't just for bodybuilders. It's actually a major part of both our recovery and our muscle efficiency, and arguably the most important of the three macronutrients, albeit the one that is often overlooked in contemporary food conversations. When talking about high-fat or high-carb diets, protein remains a constant, regardless of who is arguing about what your body needs.

Protein is made up of amino acids, some more necessary to proper body function than others, and it's what keeps us moving, repairs our tissues, and regulates our hormones.

There are 9 essential amino acids—meaning those that need to be obtained by food—and 11 nonessential ones, which are manufactured in the body. If you've heard the term *complete protein*, it simply means a food that contains all 9 essential amino acids. While this is often cited as a problem for vegetarians, since most complete proteins exist in animal sources, most nutritionists and dietitians, including Nanci Guest, MSc, RD, CSCS, believe that as long as you eventually take in the complementary amino acids—within 24 hours—it's not a problem to split them up.

"One of the goals for anyone who's exercising or training most days of the week is muscle recovery every day," says Guest. "After a workout, you're not really recovered for 72 hours, and if it's a really strenuous workout, you can be sore for 4 to 5 days after that."

We've all been on that century ride. The good news is that with proper post-ride nutrition, while you're still likely to be sore, you can mitigate some of the soreness and help your body recover even stronger. Not recovering properly can cause you to actually step backward in your progress. "If you're training for more than just fitness, even if you're not sore, you do need 3 days to fully recover," Guest explains. "Each day, you're recovering from a workout that was a couple days prior, so you're doing some kind of recovery or adaptation 7 days a week."

That rest day you took? You're still working

to fix damage you did 2 days before. So even when you're hanging out on the couch, your body is working by trying to repair. Proper nutrition on rest days can help your body repair and allow you to recover stronger. A rest day isn't an excuse to eat doughnuts and ignore good nutrition—save the junk calories for the days your body can use some extra.

For proper recovery, "protein becomes a priority, and it's something that gets overlooked often by endurance athletes," continues Guest. "It's been emphasized for bodybuilders at the gym, making sure they can gain size or strength. And even though that's not the goal of endurance athletes, you're still getting stronger, even if you're not getting bigger."

Recovery is key because "there's a lot of damage caused by a hard session, whether it's

## WHAT ABOUT THE VEGANS?

Vegan athletes may have the toughest time balancing nutrients, but it's far from impossible. In fact, vegan athletes are lucky in that their saturated fat intake tends to be much lower just by eschewing all animal products, while omnivorous athletes need to focus on finding leaner cuts of meat and healthy dairy options.

"We have gold medal Olympians who are vegans. All kinds of diets can work as long as you stick to basic principles," says Nanci Guest, MSc, RD, CSCS. But vegans do need to check their protein grams to make sure that they're getting enough. "If you're building a house and have the frame there, but you don't have the bricks, you can't do anything. You can't build, and you can't repair," explains Guest. "Those bricks in the bloodstream are the amino acids, and you need to provide that frequently."

Vegan protein doesn't mean faux meat products that are highly processed and full of chemicals. Rather, opt for natural options like legumes, nuts, and soy. Just be sure to enjoy them in smaller quantities.

"There's not enough education that protein exists outside of meat sources," says Mo Bruno Roy, retired pro cyclocrosser and longtime vegan. "But I think the more you know of protein that exists outside of meat sources, the better you can check how much of it you're eating."

As a vegan, you need to be even more on top of your food choices. It's important to keep a food diary for a few days every so often to make sure that you're getting enough protein each day. As we have learned, protein is key to athletic success and muscle repair.

hills, intervals, or just a hard ride," she says, adding, "you're not necessarily looking for hypertrophy or muscle growth, you're looking to recover those slow-twitch fibers. You have to repair that muscle tissue. It's not like endurance athletes aren't using muscles."

We also need protein to increase mitochondria in our cells. "The more mitochondria you have, the more aerobic capacity you have," Guest explains. "A lot of goals with training are about increasing mitochondria. What we want people to do is to get out of a catabolic state. That's what happens at night: The body is still trying to repair muscle, improve immunity, build and remodel bone—everything that's required for the body to remain stable and achieve homeostasis—in addition to recovering from exercise. That requires protein."

And that's why protein is so important: Yes, it aids recovery, but it also provides the building blocks to growing mitochondria, which, in turn, leads to increased aerobic capacity. And doesn't every cyclist want that?

## HOW MUCH DO I EAT?

Simply put? According to the International Society of Sports Nutrition (ISSN), 0.64 to 0.91 grams of protein per pound of body weight per day for athletes. Another way to think of it is 6.4 to 9.1 grams of protein for every 10 pounds of body weight. For a 125-pound female, for example, that would mean between 80 and 113 grams

per day, while a 175-pound male would need between 112 and 159 grams—so a high-protein day might mean some extra protein-heavy snacks during the day. (The ISSN uses the ratio 1.4 to 2.0 grams of protein per kilogram of body mass, but all ratios have been converted to pounds for simplicity.)

High-protein meals contain 15 to 20 grams of protein for the average cyclist. A 125-pound racer will need closer to 15 grams, while a 175-pound rider needs about 20 grams, possibly a few more.

While overall daily intake of protein is important, it is essential to consume protein at regular meals throughout the day, rather than 80 grams at dinner while ignoring it the rest of the day. "People should have protein for three to four meals a day: breakfast, lunch, dinner, and possibly at bedtime," says Guest.

"That's the biggest problem with a lot of people: They have 10 grams of protein at breakfast, 10 at lunch, a few for a snack, and then 50 grams with dinner," she continues. "And your body can't assimilate that. We need the protein dose frequently, and we need to make sure we hit the threshold of about 20 grams."

Admittedly, 20 grams of protein isn't always easy to sneak into a meal: For breakfast, that's three eggs, along with some veggies. But protein also exists in plenty of plant sources. A gram here and a gram there—as long as you just take a bit of time to plan out your meal, hitting a target of 20 grams isn't unachievable: You don't need a Porterhouse for breakfast!

If weight loss is your goal, don't reduce your protein intake: Instead, focus on lowering carbohydrate and fat intake while leaving protein at this recommended level. "You manipulate fat or carbs, but protein stays the same," says Guest. You need 6.4 to 9.1 grams of protein for every 10 pounds of body weight per day overall. According to the ISSN, how much protein you eat should be chosen based on how intense your exercise was that day. On hard workout days, you should aim for the top end of the spectrum, while the lower end is fine for recovery days if you are trying to drop weight.

"Carbohydrates, depending on what your goals are, can go lower if you're looking for weight loss, and add some for maintenance or gain," Guest says. But if you don't want to leave out carbs, don't worry. Protein isn't the only thing that can convert to muscle: "Carbohydrates will make muscle if you're training, they won't just make fat."

## SKIP THE PRE-RIDE PROTEIN

While every meal should ideally contain that heavy dose of protein to flip the anabolic switch, that doesn't mean you should eat protein right before a workout, even if increasing muscle mass is your goal. "For someone trying to maintain weight or gain muscle, you may want to go as high as five meals per day with 15 to 20 grams of protein," says Guest. The caveat is that you should not eat a meal with that amount of protein closer than 2 hours before exercising.

"A lot of people think eating protein means that you won't risk burning through muscle protein," she explains, "but, really, as long as you have carbs available, your body won't go into gluconeogenesis [using protein for fuel]. Those carbs will be protein-sparing, essentially."

It is important to restock glycogen stores and add a small amount of protein before exercise, but not so much that you upset your stomach and spend more effort working on digestion than you absolutely must. "If you want to get up and train without having a lot of protein in your stomach, you should still have a bit of protein," says Guest. "You won't hit that anabolic threshold with a small amount, but it's good to have some protein before exercise, in addition to some carbs that will be easy to digest."

If you exercise on an empty stomach (fasted state training) or you exercise with just some carbohydrates in there, you'll be fine. "Very little protein is utilized for energy during rest and exercise," explains Alexa McDonald, RD, CDN. "In fact, the body's main source of energy during these periods is carbohydrates. Carbohydrates are the body's most preferred fuel source as they are more easily broken down and provide the body with more bang, or energy for that matter, for its buck . . . a big advantage in all endurance sports."

# DON'T PANIC ABOUT PROTEIN

Most cyclists panic about the idea of bulking up from strength training and eating too much protein. But there's nothing to be scared of: Unless you're really putting effort into getting bigger and taking in lots of extra calories, you'll tone, not grow.

"Lowered risk of injury, higher anaerobic threshold, faster speed: Everything improves when you add weight training," says Nanci Guest, MSc, RD, CSCS. "Athletes—especially cyclists—need to understand that strength training doesn't mean bulking up, and a lot of that comes down to diet."

If you're weight training, just keep a closer eye on those calories in and calories out if you're really nervous about packing on muscle. (Although it must be said, unless you're a Tour de France hopeful trying to stay as skinny as possible to make climbs easier, some lean muscle all over is not a bad thing!)

"Someone who does strength train will tighten up and tone up without getting bulky as long as his or her diet is in check," Guest explains. "Of course, if you go hard on the weights and eat like a horse, you're going to bulk up. But that takes a lot of effort. Unless you're training to get bigger—training muscles in isolation with a lot of sets—you're not likely to get bigger, and even then, a very small percentage of people are genetically capable of really bulking up," she adds.

It's harder to convince cyclists that a protein-heavy diet (or even some added muscle) isn't a bad thing. Cycling coach Peter Glassford recalls, "I had a roadie who was having a hard time making it through stage races. When we looked at his diet, he was eating high carb and very little fat and protein. And while he was really light, he wasn't hitting performance objectives at all."

So even though you may be at what you consider the ideal racing weight, if your power numbers aren't improving, it may be time to tweak your nutrient ratios to allow for a bit more protein. If that addition comes with a bit more lean muscle, you may be pleasantly surprised, because that may be muscle your body desperately needs to get to the next level of your training and to improve your overall health.

If you're contemplating adding weight training to your regimen, simply be more aware of your daily intake, but don't skimp on the protein to avoid bulk.

# WHAT'S THE DEAL WITH LEUCINE?

Leucine is the tough guy of the branched chain amino acids (BCAA). It's the most important one for muscle growth and adaptation, and it's arguably the most important for athletes to include in their daily consumption.

"We know leucine is the strongest stimulator of protein synthesis, both building and repairing," says Nanci Guest, MSc, RD, CSCS. Again, there's that word: *building*. Don't panic. "A lot of people get worried about building, but that's just part of repair. And there are those mitochondrial proteins, and they improve endurance. Your slow-twitch fibers need repair. And you can get stronger, denser muscle without getting bulkier."

Leucine is highest in whey and, Guest explains, "whey and milk seem to be the best sources. Skim milk gives the same benefits as whey protein powder. And for vegans, if you use plant proteins with supplementary fermented leucine, that's fine as well." Those plant proteins can include soy as well as most legumes, so opt for one of those sources in recovery.

According to the International Society of Sports Nutrition (ISSN), an active 125-pound individual should ingest roughly 2.5 to 2.8 grams of leucine per day. For the 125-pound person above, that is roughly 2.5 grams per day, and more may be preferable for more active individuals. Guest recommends around 2.8 grams for cyclists.

"It's fine to have protein within an hour after a workout, but don't stress if you don't," says Guest. But if you have missed the just-after-workout window and you want to make sure you get your protein in, she adds, whey protein gets into muscles the fastest. But check the quality of the whey protein by looking at the amount of leucine that it contains. "The trick to telling is the breakdown on the label, and if you're not getting 2.8 grams of leucine in a 25-gram serving, it's not whey—they've

## WHAT ABOUT PROTEIN FOR RECOVERY?

In sports nutrition, a protein recovery shake is one of the most cliché meals. You come in from a workout and go straight to your blender where you toss together some water and protein powder, or for the hard-core Rocky fans out there, a few raw eggs.

That's not exactly what we're going for here.

Adding some protein to your post-workout meal or snack is a good idea, but you can give spiked the protein with inferior protein sources."

The biggest hint that a protein powder isn't all it's built up to be? Cost. "If you're finding cheap protein powder, it's likely been nitrogen spiked," explains Guest. "And that's why you can't go wrong with real food. Sub in skim milk instead, or even soy milk. You don't have to go after special powders." While whey protein is absorbed into muscles the fastest, skim milk comes in as a close second, says Guest. You can also find leucine in lean meats, egg whites, and most fish.

Supplements and protein powders aren't always ideal: Drinking a glass of protein powder mixed with water is nowhere near as filling or satisfying as sitting down to an egg-white omelet or a chicken breast on top of a delicious salad. "I always recommend food above supplements," says nutritionist Jordan Dubé, MS. "Ultimately, protein powder is ground-up something that's then put in water. I'm a huge fan of whole foods and putting something in your body that you recognize. Real food above everything else, always."

Sometimes, a protein-powder recovery shake with frozen berries, or a glass of skim milk with a carbohydrate source like a banana, can be an easy way to get your protein in quickly post-ride. This way, you have time to calm down and cook a good meal a couple of hours later. Unless you're training again in the next 24 hours, you have a bit more time to get in those recovery calories.

Last, if you can only get leucine in supplement form by way of BCAA supplements or whey protein, don't panic—BCAAs are actually one of the few worthwhile additions to your supplement collection. While whole foods are ideal, supplemental protein is a safe and convenient method of ingesting protein, according to the ISSN.

the shake a pass if you have time to sit down to a meal with real, whole-food proteins and some carbohydrates. Consuming protein post-workout can potentially aid in faster recovery, as well as help keep you slimmer, according to the ISSN. It is not necessary to consume protein immediately after exercise for adequate recovery, but your next meal should feature a good source of protein.

But don't think you can get away with just the powder mixed in water for the protein to start working: Protein isn't going to take you very far if that's all you consume post-ride. If you have been in the saddle for more than an hour, your glycogen stores need to be refilled through a combination of protein and carbohydrates. "Protein is essential for building and repairing muscles, as well as other indispensable processes in the body," explains McDonald. "Often, athletes think they need to load up on protein—and only protein—to build muscle. But building muscle comes from resistance-training that's paired with a well-balanced carbohydrate-based diet containing ample, but not excessive, amounts of protein to fuel your workouts and muscles.

"With this type of diet," she continues, "carbohydrates are utilized to replenish glycogen stores, while dietary protein is reserved to build and repair muscles. Muscles can suffer when athletes don't take this combination into consideration, such as when protein powders are mixed with water."

Doesn't a protein smoothie mixed with some frozen fruit and a banana sound better than water and protein powder in a glass?

## YOUR FIVE TAKEAWAYS

1. Protein is essential to the recovery process and is a cornerstone to a healthy diet.

2. Feel free to play with fat and carbohydrate ratios, but protein must remain a constant.

3. Eat protein with every meal and aim for 15 to 20 grams.

4. Adjust your protein consumption to fuel your day: A recovery day means you can opt for the lower end of the protein scale.

5. Avoid taking in protein directly before training, as it may not sit well in your stomach.

# CHAPTER FOUR

# CARBOHYDRATES

Carbohydrates aren't the work of the devil.

Sure, they're in all those fun-but-bad things like doughnuts and nacho chips, but they're also in fruits, veggies, and, of course, whole grains. And we need them.

In fact, our brains and bodies can't function without carbs, and even the most steadfast high-fat proponents will concede that a person can't live on fat alone. Carbs are our primary fuel source, and the easiest source for our bodies to metabolize, especially during exercise. Carbs come in two forms: simple (think sugars like fructose and glucose) and complex (think starches like potatoes). It's not a surprise that simple carbs are often thrown under the bus when talking about what's bad for us.

While some may debate the necessity of carbs, currently, the U.S. Department of Agriculture (USDA) recommends that adults get 45 to 65 percent of their daily caloric intake from the macronutrient. While this exact ratio can be debated on an individual basis, the necessity of the sugars can't.

To get scientific for a second, "carbohydrates are utilized for the production of glucose (immediate energy in the blood) and glycogen (stored energy in the muscles and liver), whereas dietary fat intake contributes to long-term energy storage in fat tissue," Alexa McDonald, RD, CDN, explains.

Our bodies hang on to carbs in the form of glycogen stores—about 400 grams on average daily, for someone who isn't carb loaded or carb depleted after exercise—and that's how we can ride longer before needing to refill those stores. Of course, the exact amount we store is highly individualized, but generally, it is enough to fuel roughly an hour of training.

Despite the need for carbs, there are still naysayers who want to blame one macronutrient for everything. "What is it that people hate so much about carbs?" wonders Nanci Guest, MSc, RD, CSCS. "It's not like high fat has been the answer to a million things. People don't understand that without insulin, the hormone that allows us to utilize sugar, we would die.

## WHAT ABOUT GLUTEN?

The gluten-free craze is everywhere these days. And yes, some people absolutely should avoid it: those with celiac disease. Celiac doesn't just mean your tummy hurts when you have too many servings of pasta. It's a genetic condition where eating gluten triggers an immune response in your small intestine. While celiac diagnoses are becoming more and more common, the number of people who believe that they are gluten intolerant is rising even faster. If you truly believe that gluten (found primarily in flour) is causing you to have severe stomach issues, check with your doctor.

Alternatively, some people choose to avoid gluten just because doing so makes them feel better.

Just be smart about it.

"The only people who need to follow a gluten-free diet are those with celiac disease and people who have, or suspect they have, non-celiac gluten sensitivity, which is the standardized term," explains nutritionist Jeanne Walsh Smith, RDN, LDN, RYT. However, this is where it gets a bit complicated. "Unlike celiac disease, there is no validated biomarker to identify non-celiac gluten sensitivity," she adds. "It is a diagnosis of elimination and speculation."

There's no reason you need to eat gluten, and in fact, cutting it out can lead to a more whole-foods-oriented diet, since you can replace those grains with sources like vegetables and nutrient-dense potatoes and

---

The carbohydrates don't make you insulin-insensitive, and it's not like if you take out carbs, you stop releasing insulin. You release plenty of insulin when you eat protein. But people out there with bits of information taken out of context can have such conviction."

So if you've been terrified of carbs and surviving on water and protein powder on rides, it's time to make that mental shift toward embracing the power of carbs—and that can even mean downing a good dose of sugar, as long as it's timed correctly.

"In addition to being a primary fuel source, carbohydrates are important to anyone training. For example, males who want to make sure that they have the testosterone that they need for muscle growth," says Guest. Carbohydrates are essential for testosterone production. "That's something we see in studies—people on high-fat diets negatively affect their hormones. There are increases in cortisol (the stress hormone), in particular. Increases in cortisol will blunt the proliferation of immune cells. And cortisol is also related to fat being deposited

squash. Of course, it's certainly possible to still eat a terrible diet even if you eliminate gluten. Similar to a vegan chowing down on tons of processed soy-based meat replacement products, simply opting for the gluten-free packaged version of everything won't yield positive results.

"If someone wants to avoid gluten, they can do that in a healthy way, but what's important is that they don't default to gluten-free packaged foods," explains Nanci Guest, MSc, RD, CSCS. "Gluten-free packaged foods like bread and cookie and pancake mixes are just garbage. There are thousands of gluten-free products, and 95 percent of them are garbage. You don't want to move to that processed food think-ing that it's healthy—because it isn't. It just has a bit of a health halo right now.

"When food products are labeled 'gluten-free,' it may lead some to believe that gluten is a bad food or harmful in some way," Smith adds. "It is not. Gluten-free foods are not healthier and will not promote weight loss."

Like any fad diet, it's easy to fall into the trap of thinking a gluten-free stamp is a free pass to a healthy meal. But pass on that gluten-free cupcake (it's, in all likelihood, all highly-processed sugar and covered in a mountain of icing) and instead opt for a sweet potato with some organic peanut but-ter: That's how you make a gluten-free diet healthy.

around the middle [the abdominals], regardless of what's happening in the diet." A side note: Poor sleep habits, such as getting under 6 hours of shut-eye per night, can also raise cortisol levels. (More on that in Chapter 15.)

Carbs are key to high performance, especially during bursts of hard and short efforts. It may be possible to perform ultra-endurance on a high-fat diet, but when it comes to a criterium or cyclocross race, you need those glycogen stores to get you through the race at a fast pace. "During endurance or aerobic exercise, the body pulls energy from glycogen stores," McDonald explains. "However, as intensity increases, the ratio of carbohydrate to fat burned will increase. This occurs because energy can be made avail-able from glycogen at a faster rate."

This is why taking in carbs regularly—pre-ride or in-ride—is key. They get used up, and if you've ever bonked and experienced the grumpy sensation that you hate everything—your ride partners, your bike, your helmet, your stupid socks—you've depleted your glyco-gen stores. This makes you an unpopular riding buddy and a worse cyclist, but it is completely preventable.

"In comparison to fat stores, glycogen stores are limited, and athletes will hit the wall when these stores begin to run low," says McDonald. "Low muscle glycogen stores and low blood glucose levels are associated with fatigue during longer exercise."

So if you're starting to feel rundown on a ride, it's not bacon or a whey protein shake that your body needs to power up that next hill: It's carbohydrates, and fast.

## WHAT CARBS SHOULD I HAVE?

We've been taught that there are good carbs and bad carbs. Good carbs are fruits and vegetables; bad carbs are simple sugars. But as athletes, there's hope: If utilized properly, those bad carbs aren't so bad after all.

The primary ingredient in nearly every gel, sports drink, or gummy snack on the market is some type of simple sugar. "Those sports drinks and gels are garbage carbs," admits Guest. "But they serve an important purpose in training. However, what that means is that you don't want to have them at other times. You don't want to have extra sugars or honey outside of workouts: You want to use them as a training aid, or maybe as an occasional treat."

Outside of training, try to give those sugars a break. When not timed properly, they revert to being those bad carbs again. "When you're not training, you want to focus on healthier carbs. You know what those are: natural, whole foods," says Guest.

Carbohydrates are arguably the only true low-calorie food. "Any food high in water and fiber is going to have a lower caloric density," Guest says, "and that only comes in the form of carbohydrates! Fat has almost no water, and protein has a bit, but nothing compared to carbs.

"There are fewer carbs in vegetables than in fruit, and those are lower than carbs in grains and starches," she adds. Grains are actually not pure carbohydrates, especially in processed form, since they often contain fat and protein. If you're eating most of your carbs off the bike, you want to focus on getting protein on top of those vegetables versus adding huge helpings of pasta.

"It's not necessarily good versus bad, though: Anything processed, we should eat less of," Guest adds. "Aim to get carbs from a natural, minimally processed state outside of training." The one major benefit to eating off-bike carbs in their fruit-and-vegetable forms is fiber. It may come as a surprise to some people to find out that fiber is, in fact, a carbohydrate, albeit an indigestible one. However, for a properly functioning intestinal system (and a way to ensure better bowel movements), fiber is a necessity. If you've ever gone a day or two without fruits or vegetables and found yourself a bit backed up, a lack of fiber is likely the reason why. An added bonus: Diets high in fiber have been shown to lead to lower risks for obesity.

For vegans and gluten-free folks eating diets high in fiber, it's not a surprise that having enough fiber in your system keeps everything moving. But even with those diets that you'd assume would be healthy, there's plenty of room for error.

Retired pro cyclocrosser Mo Bruno Roy has seen plenty of vegetarians who are convinced that something is missing in their diets, but rather than an animal protein, she believes that what is missing is actually fiber. Strange if you imagine vegetarians as only eating salads. "I think someone who's not eating a clean diet as a vegan or vegetarian should first try to clean it up and eliminate processed foods before switching to a different diet, to see if that improves overall health and digestion," she says. "Especially having an increase in fiber! A lot of people think it's a huge detriment

## NO EXCUSES FOR SKIMPING ON FRESH FOOD

One complaint that nutritionists often hear (and athletes will readily admit to claiming) is that during winter months, fruit and vegetables available at the store just aren't that great, or they're expensive since they were shipped in from warmer climates. Still, that's not an excuse to give your fruit smoothie a pass: It just takes a bit of forward thinking.

"Not eating fruits and vegetables because you can't get them fresh in the winter months will never be good for you. Getting them in frozen form is fine," says Nanci Guest, MSc, RD, CSCS. "At the end of the day, any plant-based food is giving you a really concentrated dose of nutrition. The nutritional value is either a 9 out of 10 or a 10 out of 10. They're just packed with nutrients."

Guest has a tip for those who crave tasty fruits all year: "If you want to make sure you have year-round good nutrition, and you're a bit of a foodie, you can try freezing your own fruits for winter during the summer. It's economical to freeze raspberries, strawberries, and blueberries when they're in season! Then, use them in smoothies or microwave them for your cereal or mix them in with your oatmeal."

It's easy to throw berries into a bag and stash it in your freezer, and if you're really serious, consider getting a second freezer (readily available secondhand for next to nothing) and stashing it in your basement to keep goodies like frozen berries and leftovers for easy eating.

because it's really harsh on the system at first, and you get bloated. But once it starts working, you get that clean, rapid digestion, and it's great. You get used to it quickly."

"Fiber aids with digestion, helps with weight loss, and helps prevent gastrointestinal diseases," says nutritionist Jordan Dubé, MS. "It's important. You need fiber in a healthy diet."

Pro road racer Janel Holcomb is a fanatic about fiber in the form of fruit and vegetables, which she includes in every meal and most snacks. "If you eat a lot of fiber, you know. And it's a good thing! When you miss out on that, you know the difference," she says.

However, try not to ingest fiber right before a ride since it takes quite a bit for the gut to digest it, and a stomachful of fiber can lead to cramping, gas, or diarrhea during a ride. Not a fun situation, especially if you're wearing a half-zip jersey and bib shorts.

## CAN I GO LOW CARB?

In a word, no. In a sentence, well, low carb is relative.

Admittedly, carbohydrates are one of the things you can cut back on if you're trying to lean out—especially if your diet is still heavier in the junk food carbs (white flours and sugars) that are traditional in an American diet. But— and we'll get into this more later—weight loss should never come at the expense of your fit-

ness and training. Rather, it should be a slow process that allows excess poundage to come off without a decrease in power and endurance.

"If someone is having a pretty good training volume and intensity and eating moderately but still has a stubborn 5 pounds to lose, that's a scenario in which someone might want to look at cutting back on carbs, as long as that's the last thing we change in his or her diet," says Guest. "With a lot of my athletes, it's the approach I use."

The reason, she explains, is that "we don't want to shortchange ourselves on protein, but we can cut back on carbohydrates."

Before cutting back on those fresh fruits and sweet potatoes, consider the fats that you're taking in as well. "With fats," says Guest, "we want the healthy ones, though we only need omega-6s and omega-3s. They're necessary for our health and functioning, and we can't make them. Our bodies can make saturated fats out of other fats, so if I see someone is drinking 2% milk or yogurt or eating chicken thighs instead of breasts, I'll tell them to switch to a leaner source. Higher-fat proponents won't like that, but cutting out 100 calories a day can make a difference."

If you've cut fat to the bone (pun intended), then it might be time to look at what carbs you can cut down on.

This doesn't have to mean that carbs are out completely—you're just avoiding the worst of them. "It's not a hard intervention to just cut

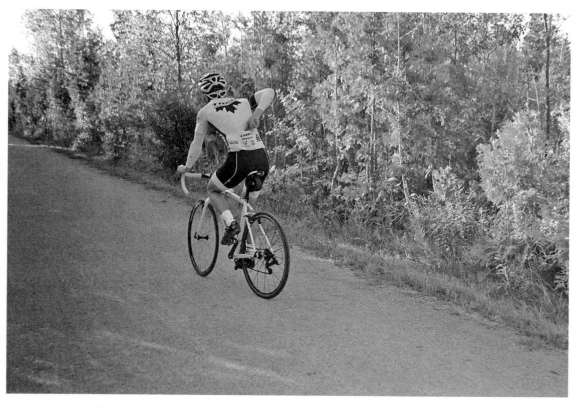

To fuel your rides, carbohydrates are king, but only if you can get your gels or bars out of your pocket!

out highly processed sugars and pastries from your day," says cycling coach Peter Glassford. "And that's when you see huge improvements. I have a client who just stops eating bread and . . . boom! . . . he drops 5 to 10 pounds just from not having those extra slices of bread, muffins, or pastries during the day. It's not that the bread is inherently bad though—it's just something that he overdoes. He's only training 8 hours a week, so he doesn't need a lot of extra calories."

You may not experience such dramatic results, but if you've done what we discussed earlier and kept a food diary for a few days to get a better picture of what a standard day looks like, you may have noticed some patterns. Maybe you grab a cookie with your morning coffee most days or have a piece of milk chocolate every night after dinner. Maybe it's a handful of chips in the car on the way home from your group ride. "If you come back from a ride and you're having a beer and eating chips, that's not going to work," says Dubé. "Even if you think you're being good about making choices and eating whole grain pasta or a bagel, that food breaks down very rapidly in the body and becomes energy right away, if you need it. Then, your body consumes and uses it quickly and you have a crash, or you don't need them and they get stored as body fat. A crash isn't good nor is stored body fat."

Removing these particularly junky choices—especially if they're choices that you find yourself making often—can lead to big changes, even if you're replacing them with

## DOES ORGANIC REALLY MATTER?

When we talk about whole, healthy foods, the assumption is that our fruits, vegetables, and meats haven't been stuffed full of chemicals, sprayed with preservatives, or packed with sodium nitrate. However, the reality is that most food isn't as clean, per se, as we might hope. So does that mean we need to buy only organic?

"There are a few things we're looking for when we buy organic," says Nanci Guest, MSc, RD, CSCS. "We're doing it for environmental reasons and for the health of our planet; we're looking for healthier food we want to ingest, and we're looking for a reduction of chemicals in our bodies and environments. So there are different goals. Each reason has a strength in it. We know eating organic is better for the planet, but whether it's truly healthier is still up for debate."

The problem comes down to pesticides. If a crop is subjected to powerful pesticides to combat things like fungus, the crop no longer has to deal with that fungus on its own. "We're seeing studies saying that there are more antioxidants produced in organic produce," explains Guest. "If an organic orange has to act as its own pesticide and antifungal, it will differ from an orange that's been chemically sprayed with pesticides. And those natural pesticides in the organic versions are shown to have benefits when eaten by humans—they act as powerful antioxidants or anti-inflammatories. There are some nutritional benefits there."

In fact, a recent study published in *Environmental Health Perspectives* shows that across the board, people who opted for nonorganic options showed higher levels of pesticide exposure. When dealing with in-season fruits and vegetables, in particular, you may notice a difference in taste when you switch from standard supermarket choices to the organic options. "Taste is a factor, too—an organic strawberry will be red all the way through and just taste better!" Guest says. A lot of this has to do with when it's harvested, and organic fruit, because it's typically produced in smaller other carbs in the forms of fruits, vegetables, or perhaps a sweet potato.

As we'll remind you throughout the next few chapters, don't confuse healthy food with low-calorie food: a massive sweet potato contains more calories than a small cookie, so that is not a good trade, especially if you're going to add almond butter on top of it. Maintaining the balance of calories in and calories out is what's ultimately going to get you to an ideal cycling body. You're not off the hook just because you've improved nutrient density.

batches, will get picked when it's ripe, and not left in dark storage rooms waiting to ripen like some modern crops. "A lot of fruits don't naturally ripen, like apples, if they're picked early," adds Guest.

Pro road racer Tayler Wiles swears by organic fruits and vegetables. "For me, it was just moving to California that made me switch," she explains. "Growing up in Utah, there wasn't a big push for organic food, but California has always been into that. Becoming more in tune with what I put in my body has become really important, and I have a lot of family who have gone through a lot of health problems, so I try to avoid processed foods and pesticides that could cause—or make worse—those problems. It's worth the money to focus on things that are organic and aren't processed."

At the end of the day, if you can switch a few of your fruits and vegetables to organic options, you're doing yourself a favor. "Even if you're not getting more nutrition necessarily, you're getting less chemicals," Guest concludes. "So if you can buy organic—if you can afford it—you should." She cautions that the problem with chemicals isn't confined to vegetables and fruits where you eat the entire thing, like grapes and strawberries. Pesticides grow into fruits and vegetables, which is why bananas and potatoes are often pesticide-laden even after they're peeled.

You can find lists of which fruits and vegetables contain the most pesticides by checking websites like the Environmental Working Group[2] for their annual list—it changes year to year, but some fruits and vegetables, like apples and spinach, tend to make the list on a yearly basis.

However, if organic options are out of your price range, don't think that this means you can skip the fruits and vegetables and feel sanctimonious about it. A carefully washed regular apple may not be quite as good as the organic option, but it still has those vitamins, carbohydrates, and fiber that your body needs.

## HOW MANY CARBS SHOULD I HAVE?

When it comes to active training, carbs are king. While you can dabble with a low-carb diet off the bike, it will need to be balanced with a carbohydrate-friendly approach to your riding. For rides under an hour, don't worry. But for anything longer than that, you're getting into territory where your glycogen stores are dwindling and you need to top off.

"You can do low carb when you're not worried about fueling a session," explains Guest. "But for athletes, carbs are a fuel—they're the body's preferred fuel source. And that means it's important to have them before training or racing, during longer sessions, and after training to replete those glycogen stores so you're prepared for the next ride."

Those are important carbohydrates taken in before, during, and after training and they count for more than just fuel for a specific ride. You're teaching your body to process certain things at certain times, which is key for consistent race results. "Your nutrition before, during, and after training impacts gene expression," says Guest. "So carbohydrates can't just be looked at as a fuel anymore."

When it comes to topping off those stores post-ride, don't panic about eating that muffin immediately. You have time. "If the next session is more than 24 hours away," says Guest, "you have time to replace carbohydrates, and the 30-minute window post-workout isn't as important, as long as you eventually replace them."

If you have another ride later in the day, or you're trying to stay lower carb outside of that riding window in order to decrease overall calories, take advantage of the recovery window immediately following your workout, and get those carbs in while your body is primed to accept them. "You can carb up right after a ride to take advantage of the increased deposition of the glycogen, because it's working double the rate for the first hour after exercise," explains Guest.

You may not need many carbs outside of exercise, but the best approach is—as we'll say over and over—the moderate one.

"Having a moderate approach to carbs allows for enough protein and fat—and people have to remember that if you're eating too much protein while on a high-fat diet, it can cause gluconeogenesis (where protein is broken down into fuel), and that produces glucose, which will take you out of ketosis," explains Guest. "So that's why people have to keep on the super-high-fat, low-protein, and low-carb diet. But then you miss a lot of fiber and a lot of nutrients. That's where a lot of these high-fat diets are problematic, and that's why people should get back to a moderate approach.

"Don't mistake a lower-carb diet for a high-fat one," cautions Guest. It's an easy mistake to make, but the point of lowering carbohydrates should be to create a caloric deficit, not more space for fats to be added to the diet. The high-fat diet may sound appealing if you're looking for an immediate solution, but as a cyclist, remember that carbohydrates are your friend, especially if you're looking to keep your high-end performance consistently improving on the bike.

## YOUR FIVE TAKEAWAYS

1. For a cyclist, there's no such thing as a bad carb, only bad times to eat certain carbs. Save the simple, processed sugars for during your ride.

2. Fill up on fiber to keep your system moving smoothly, but avoid it right before your ride.

3. Keep a lot of variety in your diet to keep nutrient density high, and make sure the bulk of your off-bike carbs are from whole-food sources.

4. Adopt a moderate approach to carbs: Use them as needed in training and in recovery, but focus on quality proteins, healthy fats, and high-fiber carbs at other times.

5. If weight loss is your goal, limit simple carbs to your training sessions, and when off the bike, try to cut back on carbs to lower your calorie intake.

[2] ewg.org

# PART TWO

# YOUR DAY

A quick note before we jump into the breakfast, lunch, and dinner break-down: The concept of three square meals a day is dead.

Everyone has a different schedule and different needs. Someone working 9 to 5 who doesn't train until 7:00 p.m. won't need to fuel the same way someone doing their first workout of the day at 10:00 a.m. does. "There's no specific time that you should eat a certain meal, because everyone is different, and everyone's schedule is different," explains nutritionist Jordan Dubé, MS. "It's different if you're training in the morning or in the evening, and every person's needs are different."

Try not to go too long between meals, however. "I find that my athletes are their most successful when they're eating something every 3 to 4 hours," says Alexa McDonald, RD, CDN.

So while I've tried to break down the different variations of when you could be training in the day and how to fuel for each of them, understand that breakfast-lunch-dinner aren't set in stone. It doesn't matter if you eat dinner foods at 4:00 a.m. and eggs with toast at 8:00 p.m. because you work the night shift. As long as your meals are tailored to best fuel your training, you're doing it right.

Whether you start the morning with a workout or a quick shower before a trip to the office, we each have different nutritional needs at different times. But there are, of course, some general rules—we started outlining them in the previous chapters—so you already know that each of your meals, unless eaten right before your ride, should have roughly 20 grams of protein and a focus on fruits and vegetables over junk carbohydrates like white bread and pasta. Fats are important as well, but the more you can get them from whole foods like avocados versus saturated fats typically found in animal sources, the better.

"Meals should start within an hour of waking up, and each meal should be balanced," McDonald continues. "What does a dietitian consider to be balanced? I believe a balanced meal is carbohydrate based—whole grains, fruits, and vegetables—with a little bit of fat and a little bit of protein. About 20 grams of protein per meal is ideal. Our bodies can't process any more than that at one time. When protein intake is higher than this, our bodies likely use it as energy or store it as fat."

And, of course, that key component to a good meal—except right before exercise—is fiber, found in the fruits and veggies that are making up the bulk of our off-bike carbohydrates. "Don't forget to make sure you're getting enough fiber to aid with satiety and weight management," cautions McDonald. "A little bit of fiber should be included in most snacks and meals. Women require 25 grams per day, and men require 38 grams." For some perspective: an apple has about 2.5 grams of fiber, while black beans have 15 grams per cup and broccoli has about 5 grams per cup.

Now, let's break down the day into the traditional meals: breakfast, lunch, snacks, dinner, and, of course, dessert.

There's a difference between being a serious cyclist focused on a healthy diet and being a fanatic about your eating habits: If you're shouting at a waitress about what kind of oil is used in your meal (assuming you don't have a horrific allergy you're trying to convey), you're just making things worse for yourself since stress can mess with your digestion and negatively impact your training—as well as your quality of life. And what we're aiming for with this book is, of course, a high quality of life from optimal nutrition that supports your training.

Depending on the intensity of your training, you'll want to shift your meals to focus on proteins, simple carbs, and complex, high-fiber carbs like vegetables. Here, we have three samples of how you should fill your plate for a meal on hard, moderate, and easy days. Fats should be present in each meal as well but used sparingly.

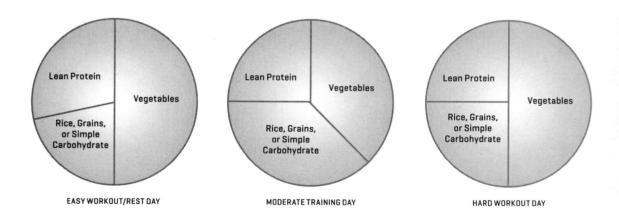

EASY WORKOUT/REST DAY          MODERATE TRAINING DAY          HARD WORKOUT DAY

## CHAPTER FIVE

# BREAKFAST

I remember being 11 years old and waking up the morning before we had to do the mile run in gym class. I went into the kitchen and, feeling very grown up, climbed onto the counter to reach the box of Raisin Bran that was sitting next to the Cocoa Puffs. This was the first morning I'd ever opted for the type of cereal that my parents ate rather than the stuff of Saturday morning cartoon fame.

I poured a small bowlful for myself, added a few teaspoons of skim milk (I was not the biggest fan of soggy cereal), and made my way through it. Yes, it wasn't as tasty as the chocolate cereal I was used to, but I wanted to win that mile run, and I knew the importance of fueling properly. Or at least, I knew the 11-year-old version.

Keep in mind that gym class wasn't until 1:00 p.m., right ahead of lunch, and there wasn't a snack break at any point during the day.

You can imagine what happened in my undernourished effort. With my stomach growling by gym class—as per usual—I lined up with my classmates. My effort was a solid one, and my result was somewhere midpack. But I felt completely drained.

The point is simple: Without a solid breakfast (or pre-race meal, in my case), you can't expect great results.

Breakfast is your chance to kick-start your system in the morning and, more important, to rev up adaptation and recovery, which was already talked about in the protein chapter (see Chapter 3)—something that can't be done on bran flakes alone.

Whether you're a morning person or not, breakfast is a hugely important part of your day. It doesn't matter if you're setting up for a long ride, heading into the office, or even purposefully not eating until your workout is done. You may be wondering what I mean with that third option—not eating. After all, isn't breakfast the most important meal of the day?

In a word, yes. However, for the sake of your riding, it may not always be a necessity. But more on that in Chapter 11, when we get into fasted state riding. The bigger issue is that breakfast—how much or how little you eat, how protein-heavy or carb-heavy it is—is like every other meal of your day as a cyclist: It's entirely dependent on your training.

"In terms of meals/snack composition and timing, I like to sit down with my clients and get into the details about their schedules and preferences," explains Alexa McDonald, RD, CDN.

"My belief as a dietitian has always been that the recommendations have to work for the individual, otherwise the changes and plan won't last. What works for me may not necessarily work for them, and that's where an individual plan surrounding a client's schedule, preferences, and training times can really make a huge difference."

## *Your Nonpancake Pancake*

If you're tired of eggs but want to keep them in your breakfast, there's a simple option: a nonpancake pancake. This one, made with sweet potatoes and eggs, may not taste exactly like a traditional pancake, but it helps cut down on your sweets-for-breakfast craving. It's especially great in the fall, since sweet potatoes taste just like pumpkin pancakes!

1 medium-large sweet potato

3 eggs

  Cinnamon (and nutmeg if you want a pumpkin pie taste)

  Coconut oil, for skillet

  Maple syrup and/or Greek yogurt

  Fresh fruit or defrosted berries (optional)

1. Prick the sweet potato with a fork and bake in the microwave oven on high for about 8 minutes or until tender. Mush the sweet potato and eggs together in a large bowl with a bit of cinnamon and nutmeg, if using, until a relatively uniform consistency. (If you have a food processor, that's even better!)

2. Grease the skillet with a bit of oil (I love coconut for this, or a bit of butter) and place over medium heat. Cook exactly like you would regular pancakes: I like roughly 3-inch circles of batter.

3. Serve with maple syrup, if using, or if you want a bigger breakfast, top with yogurt and some fruit. Delicious!

When planning a perfect breakfast, the first thing to do is to get over the idea that cereal with a bit of skim milk is the way to go. It's time to reset your breakfast to feature protein, along with plenty of lower-calorie carbohydrates to get in those vitamins to start your day right.

After you wake up, "you want the body to be in nitrogen balance with enough protein, where all the functions that need protein are being met," explains Nanci Guest, MSc, RD, CSCS. "That's why you want to have that good dose at breakfast. Unless you had protein right before bed, by the morning, you've gone 12 hours without any protein. So high-protein foods in the morning are key.

"For breakfast, even if you're smaller, you still want to have at least 15 grams of protein, in order to flip that anabolic switch and start seeing adaptations to your muscles," adds Guest.

That doesn't leave you with a lot of options, since breakfast foods are traditionally heavy in carbohydrates. "Breakfast food with a lot of protein is typically eggs," says Guest. "But it is hard to get enough protein with eggs, especially since you don't want to have a lot of yolks. But you can add egg whites—you can buy them in a carton—to a regular egg or two and make an omelet or a frittata with a lot of veggies."

"An egg white is about 4 grams and a whole egg is 7 grams of protein. So for a small person, one egg and two egg whites is great," she continues.

"Every meal should have a balance," adds nutritionist Jordan Dubé, MS. "I love eggs, and they're the perfect platform for a breakfast. There's fat and protein, and I add vegetables to get some healthy carbohydrates in there."

It's important to have variety in your diet in order to get a wide range of nutrients, especially by switching up your protein sources and your fruits and vegetables. "Greek yogurt is another great choice, but I would always suggest nonfat and nonflavored versions," says Guest. "You want every calorie to count, and if I'm looking at a protein source like Greek yogurt, I don't want the fat in there because it's saturated fat that isn't giving me any benefit. I want to avoid the calories that aren't doing any positive things for me."

Instead, make that nonfat plain yogurt into something delicious with add-ins, which improve taste, add nutrients, and will fill you up better than a faux-blueberry flavor ever will. "I'd get a plain yogurt and add a bit of honey, cinnamon, and natural fruit like frozen berries," suggests Guest. "You can add nuts and seeds to get healthier fats and calories in there as well."

If you go the Greek yogurt route, though, beware of fake flavorings and no-calorie sweeteners that are often snuck into the cheaper brands. "Under no circumstance should you get a sugar-free flavored version," Guest says. "We don't know the long-term effects of these chemical sweeteners, and we know they will mess up the microbiome and gut bacteria, and they may actually make us crave sugar even more."

Pro cyclocrosser Katie Compton likes to mix things up, but all of her options center around protein: "If I'm at home, I'll have a protein smoothie—a scoop of whey protein, a scoop of pea protein, some real coconut milk from a can, a frozen banana, maybe some coconut oil, and a bit of water and ice cubes—or I'll have quinoa pancakes or a bowl of rice and eggs," she explains.

A vegan option that still provides plenty of protein is retired pro cyclocrosser Mo Bruno Roy's favorite breakfast: "I usually eat a bowl of fresh fruit with quinoa or rice with some flax oil, chia seeds, nuts, and some almond milk," she says, adding, "that's a great breakfast with a cup of coffee."

If you can't stomach protein in the morning, or just hate the idea, that still doesn't mean you can reach for the bran flakes. Focus on consuming plenty of fruits, and work on adding protein with things like almonds or milk, like pro road racer Tayler Wiles. "My partner,

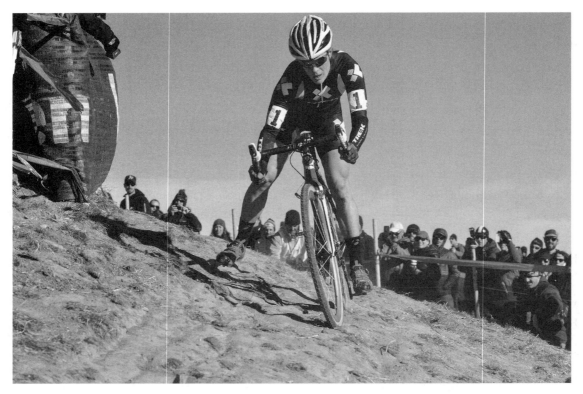

Multitime Cyclocross National Champion Katie Compton considers nutrition to be an important part of her training.

# *Katie Compton's Quinoa Pancakes*

I know that giving up fluffy buttermilk pancakes as a weekend breakfast staple can be hard for a lot of us (myself included), which is why I was so happy that pro cyclo-crosser Katie Compton was willing to share one of her top-secret recipes for quinoa pancakes. You still get a delicious pancake breakfast, but with more complex carbs and higher protein. That doesn't mean you should eat them every day, though: Save them for special occasions or as a once-a-week treat. This recipe makes about 10 four-inch pancakes, and you can use them either for breakfast or in place of bread to make sandwiches if you prefer to eat gluten-free and avoid yeast. Topping with yogurt and plenty of fresh fruit is also an excellent option.

    2  eggs, lightly beaten
 1/2  cup gluten-free or regular flour pancake mix
 1/2  cup quinoa flakes
    1  teaspoon baking powder
 1/4  teaspoon salt
    1  tablespoon melted coconut oil or grass-fed butter
 3/4  cup whole milk or 1/2 can coconut milk (slightly more if you want a flatter pancake)
    1  tablespoon maple syrup, for topping

1. Mix the eggs, pancake mix, quinoa flakes, baking powder, salt, oil or butter, and milk together in a large bowl.

2. Use additional coconut oil or butter to grease the skillet. Scoop heaping tablespoonfuls of batter into the pan (that will flatten into roughly 4-inch pancakes). Cook over medium heat, flipping after 2 to 3 minutes. Cook for another 2 to 3 minutes and remove to a plate. Top with maple syrup and enjoy.

Olivia, and I are notorious for our giant fruit-bowl breakfasts. It's always a pear, an apple, and a banana, sometimes with a kiwi or strawberries when they're in season and don't cost a million dollars. Then we pour on almond milk, add almonds, and probably put a little granola in there. That's breakfast: a big bowl of delicious fruit."

## NO BREAKFAST, NO PROBLEM

If you're not a breakfast person, we're not going to tell you to start cramming in massive meals just because it's the morning—especially if you don't have a ride until the afternoon or you only have an easy spin on tap. There's a difference between fueling properly and fueling because it's breakfast time and you read somewhere that breakfast makes you lose weight.

For certain people, eating breakfast may actually pack on unwanted pounds. "When people who don't like to eat breakfast start eating breakfast because they're told to, they often end up with a surplus of calories," Guest

## WASH YOUR PRODUCE AND YOUR HANDS

Breakfast is a great meal to enjoy fruit with the skin still on, which is why we're including this warning here. "Washing vegetables and fruits absolutely matters," says Nanci Guest, MSc, RD, CSCS. "Giving them a good rinse with warm water will help, and especially with organic, you have to watch out for things like *E.coli*. That said, washing won't get rid of all of the chemicals, because they grow into the plant—washing a regular apple won't make it an organic apple!"

To get even more gross, consider this: "Washing is also important for just getting rid of human germs from handling— that's how we can pick up a lot of bacteria," adds Guest. An ill-timed cold or flu can hurt a racer's season, so if you're a hand-washing fanatic, don't forget to make sure your fruit and veggies are just as clean!

explains. "This is because they eat what they normally do, plus breakfast. If you don't feel like having breakfast, you don't have to."

## PLANNING BREAKFAST AROUND TRAINING

For those of you training every morning, your breakfast may need some tweaking. First, consider fasted state training and save breakfast for your post-workout recovery meal (see Chapter 11 for more information). However, you don't want to train in a fasted state every day. On the days when you do eat breakfast, tailor your meal so that it is easy to digest and easy on the stomach but still contains enough nutrients to power you through a workout.

"You need to ask, 'What are your goals?' and 'What are you doing now?'" says Guest. "I can't just give a generic diet plan—I need to know about lifestyle, if you eat out a lot, how much time you have, how often you normally eat, and most important, what your training is. I have to match your diet to your training. You aren't going to have the same breakfast on a training day as on a rest day. You're not going to have the same macronutrient composition in that meal if it's right before an interval session compared to an easy spin."

Regardless of how long your workout is, if you're eating immediately beforehand, there are some basic suggestions that you should follow.

Coffee before a ride is fine—assuming your

stomach doesn't typically rebel. Some people need a bit of time between their coffee and their ride to allow for the common post-coffee bowel movement.

If you have a short, hard workout in front of you, keep the carbohydrates on the simple side and limit fiber intake to something like a small bowl of oatmeal with maple syrup. You can worry about fruits, veggies, and protein once you're finished—but don't forget about them. If you have a longer, endurance-paced ride, aim for the same protein recommended for a regular breakfast, but add in a few extra carbohydrates, like a baked sweet potato.

For pro cyclocrosser Jeremy Powers, getting in only simple, whole foods is key. "Every meal—breakfast, lunch, and dinner—is always nutrient-dense stuff," he says. But despite his rides, he's not a big eater in the morning and that works for him: "I don't eat a ton at breakfast normally because I usually get straight on the bike. But it's still a meal I enjoy a lot because I'm always hungry. Still, lunch and dinner tend to be bigger for me." If he's about to ride, his breakfast consists of simple eggs and toast. "Sometimes, I'll add fresh juice or a protein powder smoothie with fruit. Depends on the mood," he adds. His one consistent pre-ride staple? "Anytime I'm not drinking coffee, I feel like I'm a complete disaster. It's just part of the day; it feels right."

Powers is a great example—due to his limited morning intake—because he demonstrates

## TED KING'S PERFECT BREAKFAST

Sometimes, old staples are the best— like oatmeal, for example. Simple to make, easy on the stomach, and delicious. If you have a big ride or a big race coming up within a couple of hours of breakfast, a more carbohydrate-heavy breakfast that doesn't contain anything difficult to digest is ideal. That's what most of the pros do before big ride days. Here, retired pro road racer Ted King talks about his perfect morning.

"So I start the day with coffee. That's mandatory. Whether I'm going to do a big training ride or a small training ride, I'll generally have a bowl of oatmeal. That's where I have fun in the kitchen. You can tweak that whether you have your standard oatmeal with maple syrup or you put in a banana and cinnamon and raisins and apple. Basically, the blank slate is the oatmeal, and then it's how you want to tweak it. You can throw an egg in the oatmeal—that's awesome. Whether you're cooking on the stove or in a microwave, throw an egg in. You get extra protein, it gives it this wonderful custardy consistency, and it's delicious."

that it doesn't take much to top off glycogen stores from the night before in order to feel fresh for a workout. Just having something small does the trick.

Compton agrees. Her morning workouts mean a different type of breakfast in order to account for her digestion. "A day where I'm going for a run in the morning, I'll have a protein shake 2 hours before I run, because it digests well enough for me to go running and keeps my blood sugar pretty stable," she explains. But if her workout is more endurance based, she adds more. "If I'm going for a long ride, I'll do a car-bohydrate with two eggs, and then have a pro-tein shake after the ride," she says.

Since she typically has a protein shake as part of her recovery, Compton tries to avoid having them for breakfast too often. To her, shakes aren't a staple but rather a specific-workout option, "I try to do it so I'm not having two protein shakes a day. I like to eat real foods, but the shakes digest well for me—if I keep it basic—so I can go running."

Pro road racer Janel Holcomb isn't concerned with losing weight, she's concerned about main-taining her current racing weight. Therefore,

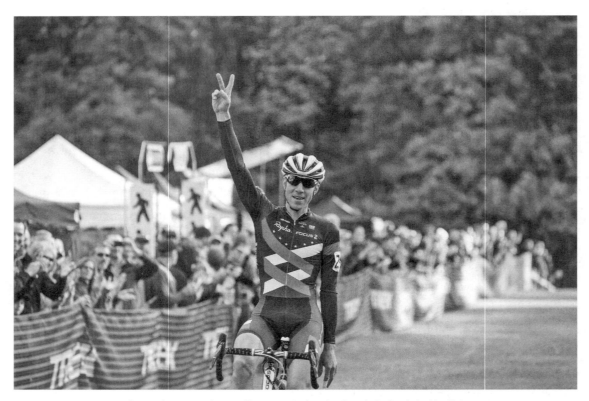

Pro cyclocrosser Jeremy Powers opts for simple, whole foods in his diet,
and clearly that formula works for him.

Holcomb consumes an almost Michael Phelps–like quantity of food for her pre-endurance ride breakfast. However, where she and the infamous Olympian differ is that her breakfast is as nutrient-dense as possible—she's found a way to keep a cereal base while still getting plenty of nutrients, fats, and protein.

"I'm strict about planning calories for a ride. Any long ride, I'm thinking about how many calories I'll burn and making sure I'm coming out ahead when I'm done with the ride," she explains.

Holcomb walks us through her breakfast routine. "I'll wake up, and coffee is my reason for being, so I always start with it," she begins. "Right now, my go-to breakfast is a big bowl of cereal, usually some sort of high-fiber, flaky cereal together with something that has a good amount of fat and protein, like nuts, in it. If I've had time that week, I'll make a muesli from scratch with nuts and seeds. Next, I'll load on a bunch of berries and half a container of high-fat, delicious yogurt, then over top, a bit of milk. That's the first course! Then I do two or three pieces of toast with cheese or maybe some jam. I find that I need the fat—so the cheese and yogurt is really important—to slow down my digestion a bit so I can feel full longer. Next, I'll add a piece of fruit on top of that. My breakfast goal is always about a thousand calories."

While you may not be planning for epic days in the saddle like Holcomb, her breakfast demonstrates the need to match your daily caloric intake with your planned ride.

## YOUR FIVE TAKEAWAYS

1. Start your day with protein—around 15 to 20 grams with breakfast.

2. Opt for lower-fat protein sources, like eggs and Greek yogurt, paired with carbohydrates from fruits and vegetables.

3. If you're training hard in the morning, start with a lighter breakfast and sit down to a protein-rich meal after your workout.

4. If you're training long in the morning, prepare for your ride by adding extra carbohydrates to your breakfast on top of some protein.

5. If you're not a breakfast person, consider occasionally training in a fasted state. (See Chapter 11 for more information.)

# CHAPTER SIX

# LUNCH

Lunch is likely the hardest meal of the day to find that perfect balance. Maybe you're working at home and doing your training ride before you eat or heading out for a ride after lunch. Or maybe you have a more traditional 9-to-5 job, where lunch is quickly eaten at your desk or at the coffee shop down the street. In any case, if you're not properly prepared for it, lunch can easily turn into a nutritional black hole.

Our goal is to not let that happen. Whether you ride in the morning, afternoon, or evening, lunch is usually the meal the closest to your ride, and that makes it all the more important to balance properly. Phoning in lunch with a muffin from the coffee shop or a wilted salad with a couple of tomato slices on top isn't going to cut it for a cyclist looking to fuel his or her workouts properly.

No time to cook lunch in the morning? Not a problem, as long as you plan to cook a little extra the night before at dinner. Almost every pro racer I have talked to says that lunch is easy:

It's just leftovers from dinner. "Lunch is usually what I had for dinner the night before, some sort of chickpeas and sweet potatoes and kale," explains retired pro cyclocrosser Mo Bruno Roy, adding, "I eat a ton of kale and broccoli."

Making a little extra chili, stir-fry, or even just making sure you cook a bit of extra protein the night before can make packing a lunch much easier. Since most of us don't have time to cook a whole separate meal, creating leftovers for lunch is an ideal solution. The best way to keep your healthy carbs up and your higher-calorie carbs lower is to aim to eat one meal in salad form each day, whether that's lunch or dinner. If you're working out close to lunch, aim to have your higher-calorie carbohydrate at that meal for optimal nutrient timing. If you prefer having your rice or pasta with vegetables and a protein source for dinner, opt to keep your primary carbohydrate source as a vegetable for lunch.

We all know that salad can get boring, so a simple way to make it more interesting is to toss an extra piece of chicken, fish, or other

# Tayler Wiles's Herb-Filled Salad with Quinoa, Cherry Tomatoes, and Almonds

Lunch is a great time to pack a salad, especially if you're sitting in an office from 9 to 5 and aren't getting any activity in between breakfast and the end of the workday. However, a simple salad can be boring and too low in calories to get you through the day. That's why pro road racer Tayler Wiles's tasty salad combines some unusual protein, like edamame, with tons of vegetables and a bit of healthy fat. "This salad is delicious on its own," she explains, "but it's also good with all different kinds of add-ins. I usually add cooked mushrooms, avocado, and sautéed bell peppers, then plop an over-easy egg on top of it all. . . . So good!"

**Salad**

- 1 cup quinoa
- 1 tablespoon coriander seeds
- 2 teaspoons cumin seeds
- 2 teaspoons fennel seeds
- 2 teaspoons paprika
- 2 teaspoons salt
- ½–1 cup almonds (dry-roasted are the best!)
- 1½ cups sliced cherry tomatoes
- ½ cup edamame
- 2–3 cups arugula

**Dressing**

- 2 cloves of garlic, peeled
- ¼ cup mint leaves, roughly chopped
  Handful of chives, roughly chopped
- ⅓ cup olive oil
  Juice of 1 lemon

1. Make the salad: Combine the quinoa and 2 cups water, bring to a boil then reduce the heat to a simmer. Cover and cook for about 15 minutes, or until the water is absorbed. The quinoa should be nice and fluffy, not waterlogged.

2. Toast the coriander, cumin, and fennel seeds in a dry skillet over medium heat for a few minutes until they begin to pop and release their aromas. Grind them in a mortar and pestle or a coffee grinder, then add the paprika and salt. Add to the cooked quinoa and mix well.

3. In the same dry skillet, toast the almonds until they start to color and smell lovely. Remove from the heat and set aside.

4. Make the dressing: Throw the garlic, mint, and chives in a blender with the oil and lemon juice. Blend well. Add the dressing to the quinoa mixture and mix well so that the quinoa is fully coated.

5. Assemble the salad: Add the quinoa to a bowl with the tomatoes, almonds, and edamame, and mix in as much arugula as you like!

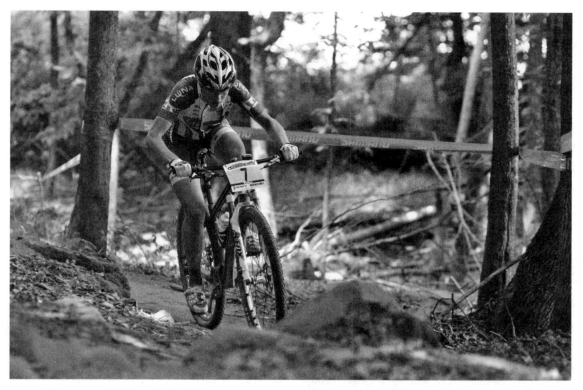

Bronze medalist Georgia Gould loves to eat and has plenty of skills in the kitchen, but she keeps lunch simple with eggs and veggies.

lean protein on the grill or in the oven the night before as you're cooking dinner. Save the extra protein and use it the next day with a mix of dark leafy greens and a dressing that won't make you feel deprived while eating. If you never feel full after a salad, add in some starch, like a small baked potato.

If you're decidedly not a salad person, think stir-fries and roasted vegetables instead of mixed greens. Personally, I prefer chowing down on a lean protein with a bunch of vegetables I roasted the night before. My favorite is a combination of sweet potatoes, asparagus, peppers, tomatoes, and beets—it's delicious and satisfying—and I don't feel like I'm eating light for lunch.

If you didn't already have eggs for breakfast and you have time to cook, eggs are also a great option for lunch that only take a few minutes to prepare.

"My go-to for lunch is some variation of eggs," says pro mountain biker Georgia Gould. "It's fast, and I love eggs. I'll do just fried eggs and toast, or I'll take whatever vegetables I have, like arugula and leftover potatoes, mushrooms, whatever, and put it in a pan and make a scramble with the eggs and veggies. I make my own bread for toast a lot, too."

Pro road racer Janel Holcomb has a similar version of Gould's lunch, often post-ride. "Lunch could be so many different things! My favorite is to cook up a bunch of kale, whatever other veggies I have in the fridge, like shredded carrots, with two eggs over-easy and two more pieces of toast or put it all over rice."

If you have a ride in the afternoon—and

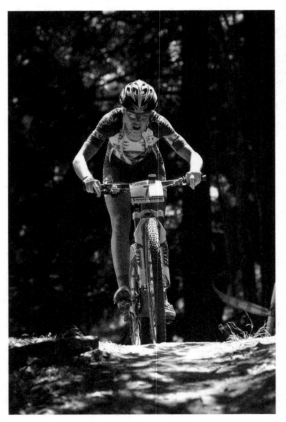

Georgia Gould is a pro mountain biker and a trained chef: two disciplines that rely heavily on perfecting your technique.

especially if you're recovering from a morning session on a double day—don't skimp on the carbs during lunch. "If I went for a run, I'll come home and have some lunch before I go for a bike ride," explains pro cyclocrosser Katie Compton. "I'll usually have some quinoa or some brown rice with some mixed nuts and olive oil, maybe an egg or some turkey."

Even pro cyclists can have a tough time squeezing in a nutritious lunch, since they often find themselves traveling the globe for racing, which means a lot of eating in airports, where the pickings are slim and the salads are pricey. But that doesn't stop them from eating well. "I bring all my own food, a whole backpack, for trips," says Compton—just make sure to not bring any foods banned for travel between countries on international trips. "I'll try to eat healthy at the airport, stuff like salads. I try to keep my diet fairly consistent." For her, consistent means plenty of greens and lean protein, and that's what you should aim for at lunch, especially if a workout isn't immediately before or after your meal.

Similarly, pro cyclocrosser Jeremy Powers makes sure that he always has staples on hand, no matter where he is. If you travel a lot, take a page from his book. "This goes to every race—I always have oatmeal, eggs, chicken, and a slew of fruits and vegetables. Simple!"

On days when lunch just isn't in the cards, make sure that you properly fuel throughout your ride and be sure to have a pre-ride snack and a recovery meal.

## TOP COOKING TIPS

Gould is not only a bronze-medal-winning mountain biker with the Luna Chicks team, she is also a trained professional chef. Here, she shares a few of her tips for getting more comfortable in the kitchen.

**Always have a good, sharp knife.** "When you're cooking in a kitchen that isn't yours and it's all bendy or dull knives, that's the worst. I generally travel with my good knife if we're staying somewhere for a while and it has a kitchen. It makes such a difference. It's not even a fancy knife, just decent and sharp."

**Volunteer to cook.** Do this when you're with friends. They might offer to clean up the mess afterward!

**Try new things.** This applies even if you're simply adjusting the way you cook the same five ingredients. "I go through phases," Gould says. "It depends on the time of year. Like, in the winter, I make a lot of stews and warm things, and when it's really hot out, I make a lot of cold salads and stuff like that."

**Pre-chop.** "I think the hardest thing about cooking fresh foods is that it takes a lot of time to chop stuff up. So anything you can do to make that easier, like chopping a bunch of stuff in advance, is great."

**Plan ahead.** "I can do it in my head," Gould

## MO BRUNO ROY'S GO-TO QUINOA AND GARLIC KALE LUNCH

Retired pro cyclocrosser Mo Bruno Roy doesn't often follow recipes from a cookbook, so her favorite meal doesn't come with many measurements. It's customizable, and—just like Bruno Roy—it's 100 percent vegan friendly. "It's super-simple," she explains. "I make it all the time. It's quinoa (or rice) with garlic kale. I just chop up the kale and sauté it with some olive oil and chopped garlic. Then I steam sweet potatoes with some beets or broccoli, if I have either. I'll add in some tofu or tempeh for added protein sometimes as well. Then I make this lemon-tahini dressing, which is just lemon juice, tahini, and a bit of rice vinegar and Bragg liquid aminos. I mix it together and put it on top. It's really simple with not a lot of competing flavors, but they taste great together. I could eat it every day."

says, but if you're new to cooking, try writing out a weekly menu plan before you head to the grocery store to avoid ending up with wasted, wilted veggies by the next grocery run. "That's the worst, when your whole produce drawer ends up moldy from unused vegetables," she laughs.

**Use leftovers wisely.** "When you make dinner, think about lunch tomorrow," Gould says. This can mean making extra and stashing it, or even just chopping extra veggies for a lunch salad for the next day. "If I have something like a big pot of chili, I'll even freeze some of it instead of having leftovers for a day or two."

**Use your freezer.** "It's great when you come home from a ride and your freezer isn't just full of almost-empty ice cream tubs or junk," explains Gould. "Instead, when you come home and need something right away, now you come home to a frozen homemade soup or chili or potpie. It's just a little bit of thinking ahead and planning."

**Buy pre-cut fruit and veggies.** Buy these, or even buy frozen. "The pre-cut ones are expensive, but if that's going to make you cook, go for it," Gould says.

**Experiment with flavor.** "The one important thing for people new to cooking is seasoning properly. I feel like a lot of people don't use salt while cooking. Not putting it on after, but putting it on while you're cooking. And also, having other spices and having a well-stocked pantry. People think eating healthy is really boring, but it doesn't have to be. You can have good spices and good salt, and you can make

delicious things that are healthy. I want food to be delicious first, and the fact that it's healthy is great. Eating healthy can be delicious. It doesn't have to be that you eat horrible-tasting, bland food all of the time."

**Learn to cook vegetables and meats properly.** "A lot of people don't like vegetables because they grew up with horribly overcooked vegetables," Gould explains. "So they never learned to cook vegetables properly. But if you can use a recipe as you figure out how to make certain things, you can learn fast. That's a huge thing." She continues, "properly prepared chicken breast is way better than dried-out, shriveled chicken breast. It doesn't need sauce or breading or deep-frying, just chicken, sprinkled with salt and pepper, cooked well on a grill can be delicious."

Cooking doesn't have to be complicated or time-consuming. There are really simple recipes out there: Don't be intimidated by what you find online, just look for easy ones. Gould jokes, "It's like, are you going to pull out this frozen pre-made dinner to heat up, or take 10 minutes and whip up some eggs and vegetables? Either way, you can have a meal in the same amount of time, but you can make something fresh and tasty really fast, and really easily."

# YOUR FIVE TAKEAWAYS

1. Don't skip lunch! You can't properly fuel your workout without it.

2. Make sure you have a good balance of lean protein and carbohydrates, but opt for more vegetable-based carbohydrates, unless you're heading out on a ride after lunch.

3. Eggs aren't just for breakfast: They are a fast-and-easy option if you have time to cook.

4. If you don't have time to cook, plan ahead and make sure you have leftovers from dinner.

5. Depending on when you ride, consider lunch as either part of your pre-ride meal or your post-ride recovery.

# CHAPTER SEVEN

# SNACKS

Snacking is an important part of an athlete's day because it goes hand in hand with a pre-ride mini-meal or your post-ride recovery. Although we're not counting in-ride eating as snacking, make sure to count any in-ride coffee shop stops toward your total daily calories!

On days with bigger or harder rides, we need breakfast, a pre-ride meal, a post-ride meal, lunch, and dinner—often with two of those meals overlapping (i.e., breakfast as your pre-ride meal or dinner as your recovery meal). On days like this, we're actually moving away from a three-meal-a-day model and toward something that resembles four or five meals per day.

On harder-ride days, it is easy to make a snack hefty enough to count as a small meal, so just be sure to adjust your other meals to account for it. "Having four smaller meals is a good option—it allows you to digest more easily because you're putting less food in at a single time," says nutritionist Jordan Dubé, MS. "The problem is that people don't have time for that.

Most people don't have time to eat three meals!" Therefore, Dubé says, "I consider those pre- and post-ride meals as snacks. So when I talk about snacks, that's what I mean: between 150- and 250-calorie meals that you would consider meals before and after a ride."

All of the pro cyclists I interviewed love to eat snacks throughout the day, but not the candy bar variety, rather they opt for nutritious whole-foods mini-meals to keep their energy up. "Midday, I usually have some sort of snack—it depends on when my training is. It may be something as simple as avocado on toast and hummus," says retired pro cyclocrosser Mo Bruno Roy. "A grain, plus fat and protein, but really simple," she explains—and that is plenty to top off her glycogen stories and fuel her rides, which tend to be shorter and intense.

Pro road racer Tayler Wiles prefers her snacks to be a combination of liquid and whole foods such as a shake with protein along with plenty of fruit. She also keeps fruit accessible throughout the day. "We always have a giant pile of fruit on the table, and we snack on it all day," she says. "We try to go with what's in season—everything we eat is organic, and buying out-of-season organic food is too expensive. We'll always have apples, pears, and bananas, though, and then add mangoes when they're in season, or berries and kiwis when they're cheaper."

Janel Holcomb is a pro road racer who has a varied approach to snacking, and as a roadie focused on maintaining her power-to-weight ratio, she tries to make sure she matches the massive amounts of calories she burns by taking in plenty of healthy whole foods throughout the day. As a vegetable lover, her daily food volume is among the highest of any of the pros (other than possibly retired pro road racer Ted King, who's massive salads defy explanation). The volume needs to be high since the caloric density of many of her choices is lower. "There are always snacks in my day," she says. "Usually, I'll have hummus or salsa and some crackers or tortilla chips, or some cottage cheese with avocado and tomatoes, or an apple with some peanut butter." She actually said the last bit punctuated by an audible crunch—she even managed to snack during the interview!

But if you want to focus on leaning out, plan your snacks to coincide with rides to get the best bang for your caloric buck. "Post-ride snacks are important for recovery, and pre-ride ones give you the energy to get through your ride," Dubé explains. "But timing matters. If you just ate breakfast or lunch, you don't need that pre-ride snack. You don't want to have breakfast, then 10 minutes later have a snack, then go for your ride."

Snack time isn't an excuse for you to eat that cookie or a bag of chips—when we talk about snacks, we're still talking about fuel. "The golden ratio applies to fueling and recovery," says Alexa McDonald, RD, CDN. "Eating meals and snacks with a 4:1 or 3:1 carbohydrate-to-protein ratio before and after exercise can help to optimize performance, current and future." Keep in mind that this ratio is not one size fit all and should be adjusted according to the duration and intensity of your workout.

A pre-ride snack to top off glycogen stores can improve your performance in a way very little else can. "Studies have shown that higher muscle glycogen levels can improve performance in exercise longer than 90 minutes by up to 2 to 3 percent, according to noted sports nutrition expert A. E. Jeukendrup," McDonald explains. "The protein portion of the meal provides amino acids for muscles to utilize during and after exercise and helps to slow digestion just enough for athletes to feel fueled during the majority of their exercise regimen."

A pre-ride snack is different from a normal meal that focuses on bringing in enough protein to aid recovery, McDonald explains. "A carbohydrate-based meal/snack containing a little protein and that's low in fat will leave the athlete fueled with limited concerns of gastric distress."

Timing is everything: "Be especially careful with eating fiber prior to exercise (30 minutes or less before exercise)," cautions McDonald. "Fiber intake at the wrong time can lead to gastrointestinal stress!"

When looking at your pre-exercise snack options, "a typical meal/snack should consist of 200 to 500 calories," she adds. "However, the caloric content of the meal/snack will vary based on caloric needs, activity intensity and duration, and dietary and performance goals."

You know roughly how much you're going to burn in the course of a ride, so vary your snacking accordingly. For a recovery ride, opt for the lighter end of the snacking spectrum. Alternatively, have a more substantive snack—between 200 and 500 calories—if you're about to tackle a monster ride and your last meal was more than 2 hours ago.

## YOUR FIVE TAKEAWAYS

1. Consider your snack a pre-ride or post-ride mini-meal to avoid mindless snacking.

2. If you're a big snacker, don't try to quit cold turkey, just switch to healthier options like fruit (for those with a sweet tooth) or vegetables with hummus (for the salt lovers).

3. Pre-ride snacks should be primarily carbohydrate based with a small amount of protein and low in fat.

4. Post-ride snacks should be protein and carbohydrate based to stimulate muscle repair and refill glycogen stores.

5. Pre- and post-ride snacks can be 200 to 500 calories, but for a normal nonride snack, aim for under 200 calories.

# CHAPTER EIGHT

# DINNER

Dinner is the time to really shine in the kitchen, and it's the easiest meal to add in those fibers and fats you were avoiding around exercise time. It's also your chance to enjoy the art of cooking and actually experiment with new ingredients and flavors—all while making yourself a meal that meets your training needs and preps you for tomorrow's ride. Don't forget that dinner is a great opportunity to set aside any leftovers for your lunch tomorrow.

Dinner is a great chance to mix up your nutrients and add in those different vegetables and flavors that you haven't tried before—and you know that if one doesn't sit well, you have all night before your next workout.

This is where your cooking skills come in handy. Pro mountain biker Georgia Gould explains, "The coolest thing about being trained as a chef is knowing what to do with different food items, how to properly prepare stuff, and to be able to look in your fridge and be like, 'Okay, I have this and that and how do I make it into dinner right now?' That's the best

thing I've gotten from my training." As a result, she says: "My diet is varied because I'm curious about different foods, and I like cooking."

It's amazing what small changes to cooking methods and spices can have on the same three ingredients, without introducing loads of extra calories. A dinner featuring chicken, sweet potatoes, and spinach can turn into so many different meals, depending on how it's spiced and cooked—Mexican with some hot peppers, pico de gallo, and guacamole; Indian with some curry paste and coconut milk; Thai with a bit of soy sauce and chopped peanuts; and American by opting to bake the sweet potatoes as fries and the chicken as baked wings with a drizzle of olive oil—the possibilities are endless!

However, be cautious not to overdo it at dinner. Our calorie needs during the day are often higher than they are at night; so by the time we get to dinner, we don't need a massive meal if we've been fueling correctly all day—especially during our rides. Although dinner is tradition- ally the biggest meal of the day, as a cyclist, you have to scale your dinner to complement what you've already eaten that day. That isn't to say that there will never be a time a standard American-size dinner is appropriate. If you train later in the afternoon, dinner can be your post-ride recovery meal, which means more opportunity to add in a few extra grams of carbohydrates and protein.

The key is to eat according to your riding. "You want to fuel your workouts," Nanci Guest, MSc, RD, CSCS, explains, "so it all depends on when your workout is. You also want to recover after the training session. Though if you're looking for weight loss, you don't want to have as many carbs, but you always want to get your protein in. If you're doing a 4:00 p.m. session and you have another session for the next morning, you want to have a decent amount of carbs as well as protein at dinner that night."

## WHEN SHOULD I EAT DINNER?

Let's be honest for a minute: How many times have you finished work, headed out for a ride, and not sat down to dinner until 9:00 or 10:00 at night? While those nights are occasionally unavoidable, the healthier thing to do is make sure that you're eating dinner with plenty of time to digest before bed. Eating before bed doesn't necessarily cause you to gain weight, but it may make you feel uncomfortable.

"In general, eating your dinner as early as possible is best," says nutritionist Jordan Dubé,

MS. "You never want to go to bed on a full stomach. You should finish eating at least an hour before you go to bed, if not more. Try to lean more toward 2 hours, though we know that's not always possible, especially with later-in-the-day training. But give yourself time to digest before bed."

You're much more inclined to eat that salad and enjoy it at 6:30 p.m. The urge to order a burger and fries is much greater if you are starving at 10:00 p.m. "There's somewhat of a circadian rhythm, where we're likely to put on more fat at night, but it's more about the propensity to take in extra calories—the night-bingers are the ones in trouble," Guest says. "It's the late-night munchers that are in surplus of calories most often."

You may also want to have an early dinner for training purposes: If you're planning on exploring fasted state training, you need to go between 10 and 14 hours without eating. That's easiest to do by simply training when you wake up. (For more information, see Chapter 11.)

You may want to break this rule and eat dinner later if you are not a big breakfast eater. "A lot of people need to have their pre-exercise meals the night before," explains Guest. "It's because they just can't get in a big enough meal in the morning if they want to train at 7:00 and get up at 6:00. There just isn't time to digest, so people get up and have something light, or have nothing."

If you're capable of making healthy choices later and can keep dinner nutrient-dense, it's not going to utterly derail your diet to eat a bit later at night. Just try to give yourself at least an hour to digest before hitting the sack. However, a dose of protein right before bed can benefit muscle recovery on heavy training days. (See Chapter 13 for more information). If you notice—possibly by logging your meals for a week or two—that the later your dinner is, the larger or less nutrient-dense it tends to be, focus on eating dinner earlier to avoid the dreaded binge.

## YOUR FASTEST MEAL

Healthy eating is hard, not necessarily because of the taste (it's delicious) but because of the time. It's easier to pick up a pizza than to make a dinner from scratch, especially when you've just come home from a long ride. But there are plenty of ways to avoid junky takeout by simply being a bit proactive with planning. Almost every pro racer I interviewed listed his or her biggest cooking secret as the ubiquitous one-pot meal. A Crock-Pot, or slow cooker, is an inexpensive kitchen tool that can make you the king or queen of your next dinner party, prepare a huge family dinner in under 10 minutes of prep time, or make a meal that can last you a week. The best part is that if you start a slow-cooker meal before your long ride, you'll come home to a house that smells like amazing, delicious food. And even if you're not a skilled chef, it's hard to screw up a stew.

Retired pro road racer Ted King uses a slow-cooker when entertaining because it's hassle-free. "In general, I don't try to wow people," he says. "If I'm going to host people, I prefer to have good food, but then be hanging out in the living room and having a good time with them, listening to music, drinking wine, and chatting. So I'll do a really simple meal, like a chili that's just cooking away in the Crock-Pot. I'm not going to invite a handful of people over to my house and be in the kitchen the whole time. I prefer to just do it all really simply.

"I really love cooking in my Crock-Pot. It's awesome, I love one-pot things that you can leave all day!" says pro road racer Janel Holcomb. "I'll braise some kind of chicken or meat with aromatics, like onions and garlic, to start with and toss in some broth or white wine, then add some hearty vegetables that can cook for a long time, like carrots, sweet potatoes, and parsnips. It's so good in the winter! Toward the end, I'll add in a bunch of kale, maybe a can of white beans, and just serve that in a bowl."

Gould uses hers to make her—and husband, Dusty's—favorite go-to dinner. "Sausage and white beans and sage in stew are great! That's Dusty's favorite," she explains. "It's an easy go-to if you have beans in your pantry and sausage in the freezer, and we have a sage plant that always has sage." It's as simple as combining your ingredients with water or broth and letting it stew all day.

While there are countless easy-to-follow recipes out there, you don't need to get fancy. To make a simple stew or chili, start with a couple of cans of diced stewed tomatoes and add in some protein (beans and/or some kind of ground or shredded meat), chop up an onion or two, and toss in some greens (I like shredded spinach) and whatever other vegetables you like. My favorite is fresh tomatoes and bell peppers with tons of cilantro. If you like it hot, try adding in some jalapeño chile peppers. Once all of the ingredients are combined, set your slow cooker to cook on low for around 8 hours. (If you don't have a timer on yours, consider buying a plug-in timer—typically for things like outdoor lighting—and set it to turn on for 8 hours and go about your day!) If you're looking for a chili-style meal and could use some extra recovery carbohydrates, cook up a batch of rice (a rice cooker is another great cheap kitchen tool) and top it with a scoop of guacamole (see "Killer Good Guac" on page 22). Total prep time? Maybe 15 minutes. Bonus: Make a full pot, even if you're cooking for one, and freeze individual portions so you have a ready-made meal any time!

## WHAT SHOULD I EAT?

As far as nutritional breakdown goes, dinner is similar to breakfast and lunch in that you want to start with around 20 grams of a lean protein source and add carbohydrates in their most natural forms—vegetables and potatoes are great for dinner—with a bit of healthy fat. If dinner is your recovery meal, you can add in more carbohydrates in the form of rice, pasta, or starches.

One thing all of the nonvegan pro racers have in common is that dinner is the main time that they eat meat, especially red meat. "Meat is not the only source of protein, though it is a complete protein with all of the amino acids that your body can't produce on its own," explains Dubé. She cautions that meat isn't an essential ingredient to a healthy diet, though. "If you pair foods like rice and beans, you get complete protein that way," she explains. "And just like with vitamins and minerals, you don't need to get all of those amino acids at once, as long as you're getting them throughout the span of the week."

Most pro racers keep well-stocked pantries and refrigerators so that cooking dinner is simple, no matter what they're in the mood for. "I always try to have salad-making stuff: lettuce, carrots, onions, some other vegetables—beets, zucchini, broccoli—whatever is looking good in the grocery store," says Gould, adding, "I have yogurt for breakfast and for post-ride, with granola. Then I have a good selection of nuts and dried fruits. In my pantry, I'll have different kinds of flour, a really well-stocked spice rack, olive oil, coconut oil, and canola oil since those are all good for different things. Then, I may have walnut oil for salads, and a couple different vinegars. Plus, a bunch of canned tomatoes and coconut milk—stuff you can throw together and suddenly you have a stew or a sauce."

For Gould, dinner is always something different, but based on the same general platform.

# A PRO'S KITCHEN ESSENTIALS

After traveling with, racing with, and interviewing dozens of pro racers, I've seen a lot of fridges and pantries. While staples vary from racer to racer, there are quite a few that remain the same.

**Fruits and Veggies:**

| | | |
|---|---|---|
| Apples | Cabbage | Oranges |
| Arugula | Carrots | Peppers |
| Bananas | Fresh herbs | Spinach |
| Blackberries, blueberries, and raspberries | Kale | Sweet potatoes |
| | Onions | Tomatoes |

**In the Fridge:**

| | | |
|---|---|---|
| Almond milk | Goat cheese | Parmesan cheese |
| Butter | Hot sauces | Pickles |
| Cottage cheese | Jam | Salsa |
| Eggs | Lean meat | Skim milk |
| Full-fat yogurt | Maple syrup | |

**In the Pantry:**

| | | |
|---|---|---|
| Baking stuff: flour, sugar, baking powder (all cookie ingredients!) | Honey | Oatmeal |
| | Muesli | Quinoa |
| Cereal | Multigrain crackers | Whole grain pasta |
| Chocolate | Nut butters (all kinds!) | |
| Dried beans | Nuts and seeds | |

"I do pretty standard starch-protein-vegetable combinations. So I'll do a green salad with arugula, carrots, cucumber, and tomatoes with olive oil and vinegar. Then I'll have chicken and potatoes or rice and fish, whatever protein and starch combination I feel like."

Like Gould, Holcomb's cooking style is simple: fresh, whole ingredients, always in stock. "I like the daily habit of cooking from fresh ingredients," she says. "If I'm living out of a hotel or can't cook myself, I'm conscious of the fact that when eating out, you never get enough vegetables. I prefer being able to pick my foods and know that I've had a huge variety of colors and, therefore, nutrients."

However, a veggie-focused dinner doesn't have to be boring. "Dinner could be anything," Holcomb says. "I eat pretty big dinners—I want to sit down with my husband and have a real dinner when he gets home from work. We do an assortment of vegetables, sweet potatoes or rice, then some protein." Her number-one cooking secret for the time-crunched cyclist? "For timesaving, I love cooking on the grill," she explains. "It's so simple in terms of cleanup, and you can grill anything!" Even if you're not a meat lover, you can easily grill vegetables and tofu. Try wrapping veggies in foil with a little bit of oil to avoid charring. The result is delicious smokiness and quick cooking without any of the mess.

Pro cyclocrosser Jeremy Powers is also a huge fan of grilling, though his specialty is burgers. "I love red meat, so I love making burgers," he says. "I think it's good for a rider to have red meat in his or her diet, in moderation. I love making burgers because it's easy, it doesn't take all night, and I can make a delicious one."

Powers says that some of the best advice he ever received was to not be scared of red meat in his daily diet. "You always hear, 'Oh man, I shouldn't eat red meat,'" he explains. "But as a cyclist, it's good to have that iron and those calories in your meals. I had stopped eating meat

for a little while, and that was a bad thing for me. I didn't feel like I was getting the calories and nutrition that I needed."

Of course, it is possible to have a wholesome, healthy diet without meat. But meat is not inherently bad for your diet, and if you're putting in huge hours on the bike and having trouble maintaining your weight, it's an easy way to boost calories in your meal.

Pro cyclocrosser Katie Compton is another pro who favors adding a bit of red meat to her dinner. "I do salad and lean protein for dinner, usually chicken, buffalo, or elk meat," she says. "We have a great meat market in town where everything is free-range and organic. I've never been a heavy dinner person; I always have liked more for breakfast and lunch and less for dinner. I don't like going to bed on a full stomach. And at night, I crave vegetables for some reason."

Her logic is something we can all take to heart when planning out daily meals: Dinner shouldn't always be the biggest meal of the day, or at least not the most calorically dense meal. "It's the nutrient timing," she explains. "I try to have more carbs around exercise and have more veggies and protein at night."

If you don't think a salad can be filling enough at dinner, think again. King is the master of the massive salad, so consider using some of his tips to make dinner less calorically dense while still being incredibly filling. "Often lunch and dinner are interchangeable in the following format," he begins. "So you get a bunch of greens and raw, fresh vegetables. And then you put whatever you want on it; put on tomatoes, carrots, sprouts. Put on protein, put on tuna, put on steak, put on nuts, put on tofu, put on beets or peas. I mean, you name it, I've put it on a salad before. When I've finished a huge training ride, it really sounds light to eat a salad, but put on quinoa or rice, have a side of bread, if you need the extra calories. . . . And then on top of that, if you saw the size of the salad I eat after a race, after a training ride, you'd be like, 'That's a salad for a family of six.'"

He pauses for a breath. "And there you have it: You're getting a ton of vitamins, minerals, and then a ton of calories, too, and good protein and carbohydrates."

For vegetarian and vegan riders, there are plenty of lean protein dinner options other than steak, and I don't just mean tofu. Just make sure you consume enough protein throughout the day. "It's really important for vegans to pay attention to getting complete proteins, but everyone else is pretty much fine," explains Dubé.

If you consume only plant proteins, you're probably taking in more protein than you realize if you add up all the small-scale sources of protein that you're eating. "People are really, really unaware of plant protein sources and aren't adding them into their daily protein load whatsoever," Dubé says. "Knowing the plant sources of protein is hugely important in understanding your total intake of protein."

For dinner, retired pro cyclocrosser Mo Bruno Roy tends to keep it simple and fairly light. While she's a vegan, she tries to leave soy out of her diet as much as possible and leans toward vegetable-based meals (see "Mo Bruno Roy's Quinoa and Garlic Kale Go-To Lunch" on page 67) with a protein such as quinoa or beans. "I do something simpler for dinner," she says. "I eat a lot of beans and chickpeas instead of soy."

Even nonvegans like pro road racer Tayler Wiles often leave meat out of dinner, though she still makes sure there's at least some protein source in her meal. Wiles and her partner and fellow racer, Olivia Dillon, are all about the veggies "Dinner is always different," she enthuses. "Sometimes we just do a bunch of roasted vegetables in a big salad with beans, some meat, and quinoa, so it's a ton of vegetables, a bit of protein, and a bit of carbs. We love cooking, a lot. When we are away, we don't have control of our food as much, so when we are home, we can control our food and try new recipes."

Wiles occasionally eats raw salads, but she and Dillon prefer to make vegetables more flavorful through roasting and other creative techniques. "We also love to make vegetable curries. We probably have that two or three times a week," she explains. "We don't put them on rice—we'll use sweet potatoes as a carb. And there are so many veggies in them

# Tayler Wiles's Quinoa, Bean, and Squash Veggie Burgers

Top the patties with slices of ripe avocado or a spicy sauce of your choice. Enjoy the burgers on their own, or use romaine lettuce as a low-carb wrap for some added crunch.

1 red onion

3 teaspoons balsamic vinegar, divided

1 butternut squash (or 3–4 sweet potatoes)

1 cup quinoa

½ teaspoon paprika

Zest of 1 lemon

Leaves from 7 sprigs of thyme (around 3 tablespoons)

1 can (around 8 ounces) butter beans (or lima beans)

2 tablespoons chopped fresh parsley

8 sun-dried tomatoes

1 tablespoon toasted sesame seeds

1 tablespoon lemon juice

1 small clove of garlic, peeled, plus more for coating

2 tablespoons olive oil

½ teaspoon salt

1. Preheat the oven to 400°F.

2. Cut the red onion into half-moons, toss in 2 teaspoons of the vinegar, place on a baking sheet, and bake for about 30 minutes (just until they start to soften and brown). Remove and set aside.

3. Peel and chop the squash or sweet potatoes into bite-size pieces, coat in a bit of olive oil, and roast in the oven until they begin to brown up and caramelize, 30 to 45 minutes.

4. In a medium saucepan, combine the quinoa and 2 cups of water. Add the paprika, lemon zest, and thyme. Bring to a boil and then reduce the heat to a simmer. Cover and cook for about 15 minutes, or until all the water is absorbed. Set aside.

5. Put half of the quinoa mixture into a large bowl with half of the beans, the onions, and parsley. Mix well.

6. Put the other half of the quinoa mixture and beans into a blender or food processor and add the sun-dried tomatoes, squash or sweet potatoes, sesame seeds, lemon juice, garlic, oil, salt, and the remaining teaspoon of vinegar. Blend until smooth.

7. Add the blended mixture into the bowl of quinoa and mix well. Shape the burgers into patties using your hands and place them on a baking sheet lined with parchment paper. Roast in the oven for 35 minutes.

that you don't really need extra carbs. Last night, we did a Sri Lankan curry with a salad made of shredded carrots with avocado, arugula, and sesame seeds. Easy stuff, but it tastes delicious."

We all want dinner to leave us feeling full, even if we know we don't need the extra calories. Most of us have grown up with dinner as the main meal of our day, so having a hefty portion feels natural. If you look at what the pros eat, you'll notice that what they may lack in caloric density, they make up in nutrient density and higher-volume foods like salads or stews.

There are a few ways to get around feeling as if you're missing out at the dinner table, while still cutting back on calories. "I like to use what I call the dilution factor," says Guest. "It's a great way to cut calories without feeling deprived. So, if you're going to use cream in a recipe, substitute half of it with milk instead. Or if you have a rich, creamy soup, add in some plain vegetable broth to dilute it a bit, and add in some extra whole veggies to make you feel fuller as well. You're just trying to make things less calorically dense, while adding a bit of extra nutrition."

If you're sitting down to a meal that includes soup, stew, or chili, try watering it down to give you more bang for your buck. "If you add water to a soup, it absorbs at the rate that the entire soup absorbs, as opposed to trying to fill up on a glass of water," explains Guest. "There's a bit of evidence that a person drinking a full glass of cold water before every meal may eventually lose a bit of weight, but generally the water is absorbed so quickly that it's not as though the water sits in your stomach and makes you feel full for any real period of time. But if it's water added to the soup, it won't go through as fast, and it will sit in your stomach and make you feel full longer."

Dinner shouldn't leave you feeling deprived, but it also shouldn't derail your weight-loss, weight-maintenance, or nutrition goals. As long as you plan your daily meals with your ride in mind, you shouldn't feel starving by the time you sit down to the dinner table—a salad should look tasty, not depressing!

# YOUR FIVE TAKEAWAYS

1. Dinner should consist of vegetables and protein with limited refined carbohydrates.

2. Try to eat at least an hour before bedtime

3. Still hungry? Before adding calories, try to add bulk, like more leafy greens to salads or more filling liquids to soups.

4. If you're not a fan of salad, try roasted or grilled vegetables, stir-fries, soups, and stews.

5. When planning dinners, don't forget to make extra for lunch the next day!

# CHAPTER NINE

# EVERYTHING IN MODERATION

Is booze ever good for you, and if so, how much? What's reasonable and what's excessive? What about pre-competition or pre-big ride? Whether you have a sweet tooth, love a glass of wine with dinner, have a minor coffee obsession, or crave salty chips in the afternoon, relax because there is room for indulgence in your diet. In this chapter, we're looking at what you can get away with while staying on track with your nutrition and training. Just because you're a serious cyclist doesn't mean that there isn't room for an indulgence now and then, as long as it's added sensibly to your diet.

"I'm a big fan of all things in moderation," says nutritionist Jordan Dubé, MS. She works with a lot of cyclists, and while she advocates for a diet heavy in fruit, vegetables, and lean protein, she does understand the value of the occasional treat.

Don't be fooled, though: A treat is likely never going to be healthy. But it can be helpful. "They're never really 'good' for you. There's no benefit to having dessert," says Dubé. "But one of the worst things that athletes can do to themselves is alienate themselves from society and their families based on their diets. If you're constantly so regimented that you keep yourself from eating the things you want 100 percent of the time, you're probably not going to be very happy or well adjusted. Then you run the risk of a full-blown binge."

Preventing the binge is the biggest reason occasional indulgences matter for cyclists, especially if you're not surrounded by people with the same goals. It's one thing to stick to a perfect diet plan when you're living at the Olympic Training Center, and it's another when you're in a house with your husband and three teenagers. "The more you deny yourself, the more you want things," explains Dubé. "If you jump into something too quickly and change your diet, cutting out all the things you used to eat in the past, your success rate might be high initially, but it's really hard to maintain. Then people get discouraged, and they go back to old eating habits, and the weight comes right back on."

In the grand scheme of things, a cupcake on a Friday is a lot better than a binge-eating session on Sunday after resisting temptation for the week. "One little setback isn't a big deal," adds Nanci Guest, MSc, RD, CSCS, "but a lot of them can start putting you farther and farther away from your goals. A person needs to think about how bad they want something."

If you stick to a largely healthy diet long enough, you will likely notice that your cravings for highly processed junk food fade away. As I interviewed a plethora of pro riders, what I noticed was that their indulgences were of the more natural variety: home-baked brownies, organic wine, locally brewed beer, and dark chocolate. None of them seek out a candy bar when there is a homemade piece of pie up for grabs. And while pie may not be healthy, if it's homemade and made with natural ingredients, it certainly beats putting preservatives and other chemicals into your system.

"I would describe my eating philosophy as pretty no-frills and pretty uncomplicated," says pro road racer Janel Holcomb. "I really like food, and I see that as a good thing. I rec-

ognize that I'm very fortunate to have a very comfortable relationship with food, and so my approach is to go with my gut, pardon the pun!" Because of that, she explains, "there's nothing off-limits. I have a natural tendency to eat healthy, but if I have a sweet tooth, I go in the fridge and get chocolate. In my freezer, I have ready-to-go homemade cookie dough ready to throw on a tray in the oven at any minute, because you never know when you'll need a chocolate chip cookie."

Dubé sums it up neatly for the cyclists trying to meet their goals: "If you have a dessert once in a while, that's important to your social and emotional well-being."

"Denying yourself all the time just makes you want things more," she concludes. "It doesn't make sense to just completely cut out everything, especially if you're not professional. If you're not a pro, there's no need for you to deny yourself 100 percent of the time. Your career isn't in the balance of what you're eating. You need to enjoy your life, too."

Retired pro road racer Ted King reflects on his nutrition choices in the grand scheme of things. "For me personally, I have something of an iron stomach, so I can function on anything. That being said, I think that you see those bad choices in the longer term. It's not that you're going to eat a bad meal and have a bad training ride. It's more like you're saying, if I eat poorly for a week straight—heavy booze, heavy doughnuts, heavy pastries, too many bakery stuffs—I definitely see that in the week to come. So if you eat really clean, really good wholesome foods, then you do see that improvement in performance over time. You see it after a week of not slipping up."

Occasional indulgences can help avoid the dreaded heavy week that can wreak havoc on your training. Here, we look at a few of the key indulgences that people typically succumb to and how to properly fit them into your diet. Then we will look at how to plan so you can enjoy some downtime in your diet as well.

## ALCOHOL

Alcohol is one of the slippery-slope indulgences. One or two beers or a small glass of wine with dinner is fine. But if you're talking about a weekend bender, well, that's off-limits if you're serious about performance. Alcohol, unlike other indulgences, doesn't just add extra calories: It inhibits recovery. And anyone who's tried to do their endurance ride after a late night of drinking knows that their power output isn't going to be terribly impressive when they spend most of the ride wishing they were at home hiding under the covers.

Guest says, "If you're going to have a beer, it's not ideal for recovery, but if you're not training for the Olympics, it's not the worst." Ultimately, she believes, "you have to be happy and live life. You have to respect the psychological components of eating and drinking as well, but you can choose when you're going to do it."

That means consider your timing. "If you just got done with a really hard training ride, don't have that beer after—have the right fuel and keep the benefits from that training session," Guest explains. "If you're serious about training, just keep alcohol away from that recovery period," she says. Wait a few hours and have a beer as your dinnertime indulgence, but don't waste a recovery window. For those beer-loving cyclocrossers (you know who you are), that translates into no post-race beer, especially if you're racing both Saturday and Sunday!

Before even contemplating drinking alcohol, make sure you're already well hydrated. "Fully rehydrate and refuel post-exercise before considering drinking alcohol . . . water and a handful of pretzels will boost both hydration and glycogen," Guest says.

When opting for alcohol, remember moderation: "One or two drinks per day for men, one drink per day for women," says Guest. One drink equals 12 ounces of regular beer, 5 ounces of wine, or 1.5 ounces of 80-proof liquor.

Alcohol is tough on the system, and there are a few problems with keeping it in your diet, especially on a regular basis. First of all, it decreases aerobic performance. "Alcohol is a diuretic that can lead to dehydration. This results in the heart having to work harder, impairs temperature regulation, and accelerates fatigue," explains Guest. She adds that it also impairs motor skills and decreases strength, power, and sprint performance. "Alcohol slows reaction time and impairs precision, equilibrium, hand-eye coordination, accuracy, balance, judgment, information processing, focus, stamina, strength, power, and speed for up to 72 hours!"

It hurts your recovery as well, since acute alcohol consumption (meaning higher intakes, usually three or more drinks) may negatively alter bloodflow and protein synthesis so that recovery from training may be impaired. Alcohol can also depress your immune function, delay healing, and cause problems sleeping. "Alcohol can interfere with sleep patterns by reducing time spent in deep, restful sleep, causing you to wake up frequently," Guest says. "Sleep is your body's time to repair and regenerate after training."

Unfortunately, booze may also be the thing that's keeping you from your target body weight. "Drinking could lead to increased body fat accumulation due to ethanol storage as fat," Guest says. "Alcohol can also act as a 'disinhibitor' to self-control, which often results in increased food intake during and after drinking and potentially increased body fat."

Binge drinking is never a good idea for anyone. "A couple of studies looking at rugby players found that power was impacted for 3 days after a night of binge drinking—meaning more than three drinks in a sitting," Guest says. "If you're out on a Friday night and have a few too many drinks, your performance might be diminished for a few days before you're back at homeostasis. You might be thinking that Monday morning is so far away from Friday night, but that drinking might be holding you back."

Guest suggests a few different tactics to avoid drinking in a social situation when necessary. First, let your friends know that you're in training, and ask them to be supportive. If they know you're trying not to overindulge, they likely won't push that third margarita into your hand. If you know you'll be drinking, be sure to eat before or while you are drinking. "Eating carbohydrate-rich foods after exercise helps replenish muscle fuel stores, and having food in your system slows down the rate at which alcohol can be absorbed into the bloodstream," she explains. And try not to start the party with a drink: Make sure you're not thirsty by starting with some water instead. Last, shots never were, and never will be, a smart idea.

## CHOCOLATE

Of the most popular vices, chocolate is easily in the top three. "I just ate half a bar of chocolate before we talked!" pro cyclocrosser Katie Compton says to me as we start speaking about

## Katie Compton's Gluten-Free Chocolate Chunk–Cherry Cookies

Even pro riders indulge on occasion, and this was Katie Compton's go-to recipe after a long season on the road in 2014. After World Championships in February, she had some downtime to cook, bake, and enjoy the off-season, and that meant making her favorite indulgence. Due to her gluten intolerance, her recipe is gluten-free, but if you're not interested in specialty flours, you can substitute the gluten-free flour and coconut flour with 1¼ cups all-purpose flour.

1 cup gluten-free flour

¼ cup coconut flour

½ teaspoon baking soda

½ teaspoon salt

4 tablespoons butter, softened

4 tablespoons coconut oil, soft

⅓ cup maple syrup

½ cup packed brown sugar

1 teaspoon vanilla

1 egg

⅔ cup dark or semi-sweet chocolate chunks

⅔ cup tart dried cherries

1. Preheat the oven to 350°F. Grease a baking sheet with a bit of coconut oil.

2. In a small bowl, combine the flours, baking soda, and salt.

3. In a large bowl, cream together the butter, oil, syrup, brown sugar, vanilla, and the egg.

4. Pour the dry ingredients into the wet ingredients and mix to combine. Stir in the chocolate chunks and cherries.

5. Drop tablespoonfuls of batter onto the prepared pan 2 inches apart. Bake for 12 minutes, or until slightly browned.

her ideal nutrition. "I love chocolate," she adds, "and it's hard for me to give it up."

Chocolate is hailed as a superfood with relative frequency, but unfortunately, you have to eat a lot of raw cacao to really reap the benefits. Guest adds that it's one of the foods that often gets touted as a superfood, but it really doesn't have any amazing qualities—other than being delicious and, for dark-chocolate lovers, containing some antioxidants. But that doesn't mean you should swap your antioxidant-rich blueberries for a candy bar.

You should never consider chocolate as a healthy option, but if you have a sweet tooth for chocolate, try a chocolate-flavored protein powder for your recovery smoothie, or opt for a dark chocolate with a high percentage of cocoa. "Dark chocolate is a good option occasionally, and it has a lot of antioxidants," says Dubé. As we mentioned before, in order to avoid bingeing, it's better to have a small piece of your indulgence rather than trying to replace it with something else. Don't scarf down dark chocolate thinking it's a healthy alternative if what you're really craving is sweeter milk chocolate.

If you just can't live without chocolate, it's okay to keep it in your diet, just limit your portion size, and remember to cut back on other carbohydrates to make up for it. "I eat a lot, I eat a huge variety, and I'm a relatively healthy eater," Holcomb says. "I eat well, but I also eat anything that strikes my fancy. So if I open up my refrigerator right now, it would be filled with fruits and vegetables and dairy products and stuff full of wholesome, simple ingredients. But there are also treats—there's a section of the fridge reserved for chocolate! I don't have any dietary restrictions, and that makes it pretty darn easy, too."

You can also train your tastebuds to enjoy other types of sweet treats like fruit. "I like to encourage people to have a piece of fruit if they're craving something sweet, especially as they're trying to develop their tastebuds back to more natural tastes," adds Dubé. "Fruit is really satisfying and sweet. Or making things like chia pudding or a smoothie will satisfy that sweet tooth."

## BAKED GOODS

Who doesn't love stopping at a small café in the middle of a long ride and enjoying an espresso and a cookie? Baked goods are the biggest downfall for many otherwise wholefoods devotees, and one of the hardest habits to break. You may feel satisfied switching out your milk chocolate bar for a couple of squares of dark chocolate but cutting out baked goods is arguably harder. "I love to make breads, like pumpkin or carrot or cornbread, and have that before or after a ride as an indulgence," admits Compton.

Pro road racer Tayler Wiles echoes her sentiments, saying, "I try to make my treats things that I eat on a ride. I feel like if you eat it only on the ride, it's not bad. Cookies are definitely my guilty pleasure."

Including a baked good into your carb-heavy pre-ride meal or in-ride snack is the smartest way to incorporate that particular indulgence into your diet—and keep your ride a bit more interesting!

"Making small changes and adjustments and truly considering eating as a lifestyle, not as a diet, is key," says Dubé. "So, moderation is important." *Moderation* is the key word here. If you had a piece of cake on your ride, make sure to balance it by cutting back on pasta or rice at dinner and adding more vegetables.

We're not talking about store-bought, prepackaged cookies and treats. Like Compton and Wiles, pro mountain biker Georgia Gould also tries to make her own treats when she indulges in baked goods. In their own kitchens, the pros can control the ingredients and avoid preservatives and chemicals. "Even what I would define as crap really isn't," says Gould. "I like sugar; I have a sweet tooth. If it means no sugar and you win the gold medal at the Olympics, then maybe the gold medal isn't for me. I like making cupcakes sometimes but I'm not pouring sugar down my throat!"

If you're going to indulge in a treat, savor and enjoy it.

"One of the things that is completely necessary when you're having a dessert or a drink is that you just embrace it," says Dubé emphatically. "Being filled with guilt when you're eating or drinking something, and being filled with guilt afterward, isn't going to do anything for your health or overall well-being. So if you're going to have a cupcake, commit to it and enjoy it. If you're not enjoying it, why are you eating it?"

## COFFEE

Some of us are coffee fiends, and while it's not ideal if your morning can't start without a cup, coffee is one of the least problematic of the indulgences—at least, as long as you're not referring to a 500-calorie sugar-and-fat beverage masquerading as coffee. If it's topped with whipped cream and syrup, it simply doesn't count as coffee.

On its own, though, coffee is not so bad. "Coffee helps hydration," Dubé says. "Anything made with water is going to help hydration status. I don't consider coffee a bad thing. There are benefits to only drinking coffee on race day, the obvious one being that if you get a buzz from it, it can help performance in some ways."

That doesn't mean you should be drinking coffee all day every day. Like most things, "it's everything in moderation. If you're a one-cup-a-day drinker, great," Dubé says. "If you're a pot-a-day drinker, then that's not helping you. Chances are you need more sleep versus more coffee."

## CLEAN TREATS

It's important to stop looking at indulgences as things that have to be bad for you. Instead, think of these occasional sweets as treating yourself. I don't mean a massive milkshake, but rather something that's healthier, or something you wouldn't normally spend money on. Reframe the argument, and suddenly, that mango for dessert seems pretty appetizing.

Vegan retired pro cyclocrosser Mo Bruno Roy

is a major fan of this concept. She actually looked confused when I asked about her indulgences.

"I joked about this the other day," she says, "And my favorite indulgence is store-bought kale chips! It's no joke. I love them, and they're six bucks a bag! But I treat myself every once in a while." She also enjoys organic, pressed juices as another indulgence: Again, not necessarily for their caloric content (though typically juice is quite high in sugar), but because they're more expensive than a typical beverage. "I just went to a juice shop that had all cold-pressed fresh juices," she admitted, "and they had this chai creamy cashew faux milkshake, but it was nine bucks. I think the indulgence for me is spending more money, not eating something that's bad for me."

When it's phrased like that, it just sounds so logical, right? Indulgences, food, or otherwise, should be viewed as a reward for your hard work.

Holcomb takes a similar approach: While she indulges when she feels the craving, her indulgences are closer to reasonable, healthy options than all-out pleasure-fests of fat and sugar. "The majority of stuff I eat is healthy, but if I want tortilla chips and salsa, I'll have it," she says. "I am conscious of the fact that I want to take good care of my body, though—I enjoy eating fruits and vegetables, and I enjoy cooking. I try to emphasize fruits and vegetables at every meal. But that's an enjoyable part of eating for me, not something that *has* to be done."

## CELEBRATE GOOD TIMES

After a great race or ride, it can be really tempting to hit the pub, or the after party, and go a little crazy. While you should certainly celebrate great rides and benchmark results, don't ruin all of your hard work by overindulging, whether that's on too many margaritas, nachos, or fried ice cream. (I admit it. Most of my after parties happen at Mexican restaurants.) Indulge, but pick a vice instead of going hog-wild.

To keep with the Mexican theme, if you're craving a margarita, have one, two at the most, but then keep your dinner relatively clean with something like fajitas where you can control how much cheese and sour cream gets piled on, and skip the dessert menu. If you're craving something salty, go for the chips, but skip the booze altogether or limit yourself to something less caloric than a margarita, like tequila and club soda with lime. And if you have a massive sweet tooth, go light for dinner, skip the booze, and save room for that dessert. There's no reason you can't indulge once in a while, but try to keep the indulgences at a reasonable level. You don't want tomorrow's training ride screwed up by a night of poor sleep from a stomach ache or, even worse, a hangover from hell the next day.

The best tip for those wanting to celebrate? Party with your friends potluck-style at someone's house or at the park where a race or ride ends. Often, you'll end up with healthier options, and without unlimited chips and the ability to order just one more round, you'll probably stay in the healthy indulgence territory with less effort, while feeling satisfied and saving a few bucks.

## ENJOY YOUR OFF-SEASON

Everyone needs to take a break from their routines, and as cyclists, we are lucky that our off-season (unless you're a cyclocrosser with a serious goal for National Championships in January) comes right during the holiday season. This allows us to have a bit more normalcy in our diets to keep us fresh compared to our stricter diets during race season.

King laughs about riders he knows who don't take time to relax their diets. "There's so much discipline that you have to maintain over the course of an entire season that I think it's nutty when you meet these crazy amateurs, and I don't mean they're amateur eaters. They're amateur cyclists and they're like, 'At the end of the season, I had a slice of cake.' And I'm like, 'You should, man.'"

He adds, "I think that's just insane—there's an ebb and flow in the racing season. If you're really picking a peak, then eat clean for a good, long while. So on the micro level, over the course of the week, have one meal, reward yourself with ice cream, whatever. And at the end of the racing season, don't count calories for a month straight."

Wiles admits that she can't keep her eating perfect all year, nor does she want to. The off-season is the perfect time to indulge and maybe pack on an extra pound or two, but it's certainly not a license to go crazy and devour everything in front of you. "It's the off-season where you have to think about what you eat, though you do need to take it easy and let go a little bit," she adds. "That's how you maintain for racing: Enjoy the off-season, and eat those cookies and cakes, and then during the season, stick to the whole foods and stay away from the stuff that you know is bad for you."

"You can't be strict all the time, or you'd go nuts," Wiles admits and adds that the off-season is ideal for her to indulge since feeling more tired on a less-whole-foods-focused diet isn't as important in the off-season as it is heading into race season. "I can tell during the holidays when I get more relaxed and my family is cooking for me. So over the holidays, I definitely feel that I get a bit more sluggish. When you eat clean, you just feel so much better!"

Off-season is also a chance to work on other areas of your life and maybe take a bit of a break from focusing on your diet. "People who have a fitness goal and work as well have it rough," says Guest. "Say you have a big project coming up and your energy needs to go to that—just let your nutrition go a little and then get stricter when you have that extra willpower

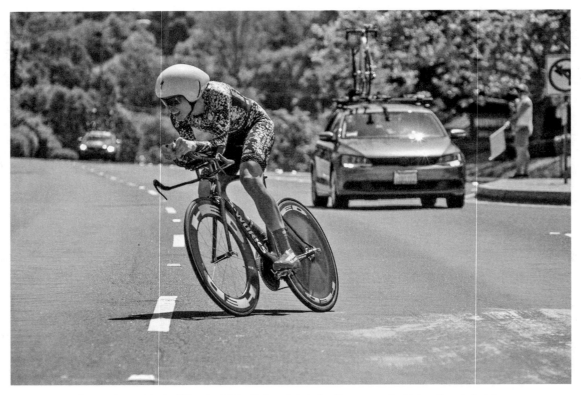

Pro road racer Tayler Wiles is strict with her diet during the season but takes time to indulge
in the off-season.

and don't have as many demands in life. When there's lots going on, that's when you get exhausted and overtrained. We all know deep inside what we're capable of. Sometimes, life gets in the way, and in the long run, it's not worth hurting your overall health by trying to stay perfect all the time at the risk of increasing your stress."

Take this balanced attitude into the season as well—just limit the size and frequency of your indulgences. "When you're getting ready for your race season and you're training a lot, that's when you need to make sure you make those good choices, like having a small piece of pie instead of a big piece of pie," says Gould. "Just try to minimize that stuff, like having an apple instead of apple pie."

# YOUR FIVE TAKEAWAYS

1. Indulgences are not a bad thing—just make sure you acknowledge them and don't make them a habit.

2. There will never be a truly great argument for the health benefits of alcohol or chocolate, but that doesn't mean you should never enjoy them.

3. Moderation in all things—period. Listen to and reasonably satisfy your cravings to avoid the dreaded binge.

4. It will be easier to stay focused during the race season if you use part of your off-season as a chance to cut loose and enjoy more indulgences.

5. Try to shift your definition of an indulgence to healthier versions of things, like fruit, dark chocolate, or even financial splurges like pricey organic juices.

# PART THREE

## YOUR RIDE

You would think a book called *Fuel Your Ride* would start with what you should eat on the bike, right? The fact is, though, that the success of your ride started with what you had for breakfast, lunch, and dinner. "It's not just about what you're eating in your workout, it's about what you're eating throughout the entire day and over a period of time," says Nanci Guest, MSc, RD, CSCS.

Acute nutrition—nutrition that's happening right now—is important (we will address that in the next few chapters), but it's really chronic nutrition—the day-in-day-out, constant way that you're eating—that plays a much bigger part in your overall health and ultimate performance on the bike. You can't eat a diet of McDonald's for 3 years and head out on a ride and assume it will go well. Similarly, making your own in-ride food won't make you any faster if you're eating pizza as your post-ride recovery meal every day. And all the sports drinks in the world aren't going to improve your time up that hill if you're drinking a six-pack every night.

What you take in during a ride might affect your ability to finish that particular ride, but everything else—the recovery and the adaptation—relates to what you eat before and after the ride. If you put into practice the principles laid out in the first two parts of this book, I promise that your riding will improve whether or not your in-ride nutrition is dialed in perfectly.

That said, what you eat and drink during your ride is hugely important to your success in the ride and in your ability to recover faster. If you're hoping to improve performance, have better races, or keep up with a fast group on the weekend, this is one of the main ways to get those extra watts, even if you don't have time to add extra training hours.

It's about finding the fuel in-ride that's best for you, and for some, that's drinking calories; for others, it's eating sandwiches. "Sports nutrition is all about the science and the individual athletes," explains Alexa McDonald, RD, CDN. "Even the most efficient and effective fuel will not be appropriate if the individual athlete cannot tolerate it during performance."

While we know that sports nutrition is heavily based on individual preference, there are some principles that are true across the board. For example, "refueling and hydration are of the utmost priority during athletic performance lasting greater than 60 minutes," McDonald explains. "A mix of carbohydrate from varying sugars, which may be most easily obtained via a specifically designed sports drink, gel, or energy bar, has been shown to be most effective in enhancing carbohydrate oxidation during exercise. Sports drinks also provide the added benefit of electrolytes to improve water absorption."

There is a plethora of other options that are just as effective when used properly. But when it comes to in-ride and in-race nutrition, remember that carbohydrates are king, and electrolytes with proper hydration can make or break your ride.

# CHAPTER TEN

# IN-EXERCISE HYDRATION

While eating on the bike may seem like the hottest topic—whole foods versus bars, getting the perfect ratio of macronutrients, and so on—what to drink on the bike is still a serious debate. No one can argue against the necessity of staying hydrated, but what about carbohydrates, electrolytes, and that terrifying problem of becoming overhydrated?

Before we can even get into that, there's one dilemma that many people—from newbie to advanced—ignore completely. Are you capable of drinking on the bike? I don't mean just taking a sip from your bottle when riding solo on a straight, flat road with a massive shoulder. I'm talking about taking a drink when riding at a tempo pace with a group, or while rolling through some singletrack. Suddenly, getting out that water bottle doesn't seem like such a simple task, does it?

When it's the hardest to grab at our bottles is often when we need them the most. Hydration doesn't wait until you're ready to sip, and dehydration doesn't care if you're pinned at your threshold on a hard ride hanging on for dear life.

The first step to proper in-ride hydration isn't mixing the perfect bottle, it's practicing on the bike. That's right, you're going to start with drinking drills. Try grabbing and putting the bottle back 10 times every ride (inside on a trainer or outside), or go for it while in a rooted section of your next mountain bike ride, or ask a friend to keep an eye on you as you try to grab a bottle while riding right next to him or her. You may feel silly doing this, but think about how much easier it'll be to stay hydrated if you can drink in any kind of ride situation! I can recall so many rides where I bonked by the end simply because I was so focused on holding on to the wheel of the guy in front of me

# THIS SKILL TAKES PRACTICE

Drinking on the bike sounds simple, but for a lot of us, when the riding gets tough, we get worse at drinking. Many athletes on and off the road that can improve their ability to drink and eat while going hard and while riding in a group. Cycling coach Peter Glassford sees this all too frequently. The cure? He says, "Practice!"

He explains, "I see this a lot with skills like drinking and eating, things that seem mundane. People don't bother to work on these basic skills in training, and it hurts them in races. The better you are at pulling your bottle out, the more you can drink. A good mountain biker should be able to pull out his bottle in the middle of tight single-track, hold it in his mouth if he has to, take a sip, and put it back without slowing down substantially."

While a 45-minute ride without proper hydration may not kill you, those epic rides you're dreaming of will have to stay dreams unless you learn to fuel properly. "In a long 100-mile mountain bike race, you may have sections of tough single-track that will take you an hour to complete, and if you can't drink during that, you're going to fade by the end," says Glassford. "So that skill may sound mundane, but it's a big part of success. The

same goes for pulling food out of your pocket. If you're not comfortable reaching around and grabbing things out of your pocket, that will hurt your nutrition. So skills do relate to nutrition, weird as it may seem."

What are you waiting for? Use each ride as a skill-builder until you're practically pro (but don't expect a soigneur to catch and refill your bottle midride—you're not that pro). Even indoor trainer rides are a great opportunity to practice grabbing your bottle and putting it back while keeping your eyes straight ahead—the goal is to learn is how to grab your bottle, drink, and put it away without taking your eyes off the trail or the road ahead of you. It's a small skill, but it makes a big difference in your riding and your hydrating!

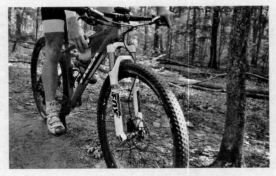

Practice makes perfect when it comes to taking your water bottle in and out of your bottle cage. Try to do this a few times each ride without stopping or slowing down.

and trying to stay in his draft that I never reached down for the bottle, and I ended up dehydrated, underfed, and just plain grumpy.

Drinking is arguably more important than eating on the bike: "Hydration is a big one," says Nanci Guest, MSc, RD, CSCS. "We can get away with a lot with regard to fuel and nutrient timing, but that's key."

## HOW MUCH DO YOU NEED?

You may think that you're taking in plenty of fluids during a ride or during a race, but unfortunately, you probably need more than you think. A couple of swigs every 30 minutes just isn't enough. A recent study that looked at recreational mountain bike riders during a race showed that 85 percent of them could be considered dehydrated (according to urine color) post-race. Even in what was described as a recreational short mountain biking race in a temperate environment with access to fluids during exercise, these riders still weren't drinking enough. It's easy to see how your hydration needs in a long race may not be met.

It's important to stay ahead of your hydration. According to the American College of Sports Medicine (ACSM), you should drink 3 to 8 ounces of water every 15 to 20 minutes—so 16 ounces (one small bottle) per hour is generally a good place to start and one that most nutritionists and pros agree on.

Stacy Sims, MSc, PhD, a leading expert on the science of in-exercise hydration, believes that how much you drink and when you drink should be based on the individual. She says, "There isn't a perfect generalization you can truly make because the link between dehydration and performance is often hazy. But, commonly, drinking to thirst for the first 2 to 3 hours is okay, but after that your thirst is not a reliable indicator of hydration. According to new research and consensus from the Institute of Medicine (IOM), the maximum amount you should drink is 800 milliliters (27 ounces) in an hour when hydrating on a schedule in a temperate environment. In the heat, more fluid may be needed. Then, you can reduce or add a bit, depending on how you feel, whether you're peeing a ton, feeling thirsty—that kind of thing."

Also you may need less if you're a smaller rider, or you may need a few extra ounces if you're a larger rider who sweats a lot. You can adjust the amount by adding more or less per hour, depending on thirst, but keep 16 ounces in mind as a base hydration level.

Weather also influences hydration status. You need to drink a bit more in the summer because you're sweating more, but that doesn't mean you can altogether skip sipping in the winter. You can get away with drinking a bit less in cold weather, but make sure that you're still hydrating. Insulated bottles help to keep water from freezing in the winter or getting too warm in the summer, so if you live in a particularly hot or cold climate, consider investing in fancier bottles. Otherwise, plan stops on rides to swap out any frozen or overheated water.

Swapping your sports drink for a heated broth is a great cold-weather option. It sounds weird, but it tastes delicious and provides hydration and electrolytes with minimal calorie additions. Plus, it makes you feel less miserable when the weather gets rotten: They do say that chicken soup is good for the soul! (Just save the noodles for your post-ride meal.)

## ELECTROLYTES

You should experiment with the amount of electrolyte mixture you add to your bottles, since individuals sweat at different rates. "Since the amount of water you drink per hour is just a ballpark, if I'm working with someone, I always have them work with pee strips to see how hydrated or dehydrated they are through the course of training," Dr. Sims says. (See the Appendix: Testing on page 191 for more information on pee strips.)

"A lot of people think just drinking water is fine, but if you're just drinking water, you're not really pulling in fluid and you can be pushed into hyponatremia really easily," says Dr. Sims. Hyponatremia is almost the opposite of dehydration, and potentially just as deadly: It's the state when you've ingested so much water that you've leeched the electrolytes out of your system. "You read a lot about drinking according to

thirst, but there are body composition and sex differences to consider. At certain points in the month in a woman's cycle, she's a lot more susceptible to hyponatremia because of her hormones. But if you add a bit of salt and glucose to her water, that solves the issue," she adds.

Guest echoes her sentiments, saying, "I'm a major proponent of electrolytes in sports drinks. Normally, your cells have a certain amount of sodium in them, but if you're drinking too much water, you're diluting it. Too much or too little can be fatal. So if you use a sports drink instead of water, it has sodium levels similar to your cells so you're adding that back in, and you'll keep it."

If you're not a fan of sports drinks, don't worry. There are electrolyte and salt tablets that you can add to your water. "But if you're just drinking water and peeing a lot," Guest cautions, "It could mean that you're actually diluting your bloodstream and have too much water. It doesn't have to be a sports drink, but even something salty—a pinch of sea salt in

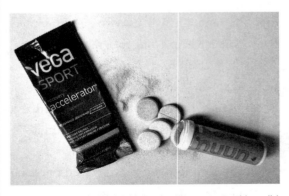

An electrolyte or caloric drink mix allows you to skip solid food on the bike.

your bottle or salt tabs—will help."

An easy way to think about it is by picturing the water in our bodies. "There isn't any pure water in the body—it's all a solution of electrolytes and amino acids, and that's how water flows through the body. So if you're just taking in plain water, your body won't absorb it well. When you start thinking about exercise, you have even more bloodflow diverted from the gut, so it's harder to pull things across. A little salt and a little sugar are going to work well to pull it over, though," says Dr. Sims.

How can you tell if you're overhydrated or low on electrolytes? Although Dr. Sims relies on pee strips for the full story, how often you urinate is also a good indication. "Peeing too much is a huge issue," explains Guest. "You think, I'm drinking all this water. But water is a good thirst-quencher and not a great rehydrator. Rehydrating means your body is maintaining the hydration. If you're just drinking and peeing it out, that doesn't mean that your muscles or heart are satisfied."

For rides where you plan to drink your calories, opt for a low-calorie, electrolyte-rich sports drink, or make your own. (See "Make Your Own Sports Drink," next column.)

## DO YOU NEED CALORIES IN YOUR WATER?

It isn't necessary to supplement what you eat on the bike with calories in your water, but a

## MAKE YOUR OWN SPORTS DRINK

When we think of sports drinks, we think of expensive powders and colorful marketing schemes. And while some sports drinks are tasty, if you're on a budget or prefer something a little simpler, you don't need to shell out big bucks to keep your ride fueled. "It doesn't always have to be Gatorade or Powerade," Nanci Guest, MSc, RD, CSCS, explains. "You can make your own."

Her favorite recipe is simple, and there's plenty of room to tweak it to fit your specific needs: organic cranberry or orange juice (the frozen mix is great if you're on a budget—but opt for the non-pulp version since the fiber in pulp can irritate the gut midride—and be sure to pre-mix with water to make juice before following the ratio below!), filtered water, and a pinch of sea salt. That's it!

For a normal ride: Mix a 2:1 ratio of water to juice, and for a lighter option: 3:1 or 4:1 ratio of water to juice. Add a pinch of sea salt.

small amount of calories in the form of glucose or fructose will help move the electrolytes through your system.

"I am all about 'eat your calories and drink

something that's going to hydrate,'" explains Dr. Sims. "Don't think about the calories in the bottle at all, that sugar in the water with electrolytes is just there to act as a transporter."

If you're not great at eating on the bike, or you have a sensitive stomach, you can take your calories in liquid form. Alexa McDonald, RD, CDN, says, "Liquid calories are a great way to stay hydrated, while replenishing electrolytes that are lost through sweat and getting carbohydrates for fuel." In fact, she believes fluid and carbohydrate needs can be adequately met through 7 to 10 ounces of a beverage containing 6 percent carbohydrates every 20 minutes. For optimal nutrient absorption, aim to consume about one 16- to 20-ounce bottle of conventional sports drink per hour. She adds, "Most sports drinks range from 4 to 8 percent carbohydrates with anything higher likely resulting in gastric distress."

When looking for a sports drink to fuel your ride, look for one that has multiple sugar sources. "The best sports drinks provide a mix of different carbohydrates, such as glucose and fructose, and have been linked to better performance compared to drinks that only con-

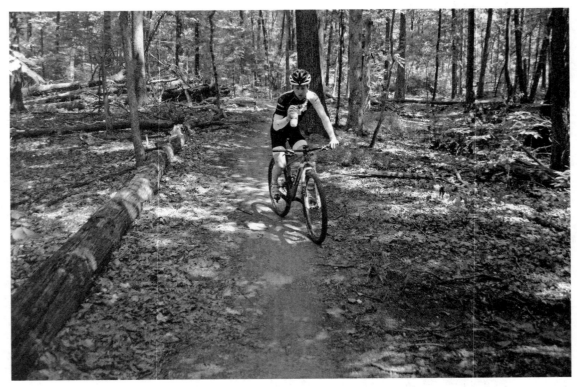

Practicing pulling your bottle out of the cage and putting it back in is one of the first skills you should work on—and it's even harder to do on singletrack!

tain one carbohydrate source," McDonald explains.

"Glucose and fructose use different transporters to get across the intestinal wall," Guest explains, "and that can be good when you're doing rides longer than 4 hours, where you need to get more and more calories in, since beyond 4 hours of endurance you're running out of glycogen stores and fully depending on outside sources. The multiple sources won't be bottlenecked at the same transporter to get into cells. So when you're going long, you want to choose sources with multiple types of sugars in them."

If you often have stomach pains, cramps, and embarrassing bathroom issues on the bike, it's even more important to make sure you're mixing sugars. A recent study done by P. B. Wilson and S. J. Ingraham looked at runners drinking a glucose-only solution compared to those ingesting a glucose-fructose option and found that, after 2 hours of running, those who drank the glucose-fructose mixture had a better time trial performance. The authors of the study believe the improved performance was a result of lower gastrointestinal distress and its psychological effects.

Guest adds that while most versions of glucose and/or fructose are fine, stick with a sport-specific formula, or dilute what you're drinking. Drinks like Snapple or Coca-Cola are so sugar-laden that your stomach will actually suck additional water from the body to dilute them. "That's where you get the nausea or diarrhea, and you can also actually dehydrate," she cautions. "You're taking water out of your system into your stomach. That's why we always dilute, and that's why sports drinks were invented." Even the recipe on page 105 is diluted with a 2:1 water-to-juice ratio.

Just as the total amount of water you need changes based on individual size and needs, the amount of liquid carbohydrates is different for each individual. "In my opinion, athletes benefit most when they fine-tune the importance of carbohydrate repletion, carbohydrate mix, electrolyte balance, and hydration to their individual preferences," says McDonald. "Athletes should play around with different mixes to see what works best for them during practice sessions so they are fully prepared for competition. The preference for a liquid and solid fuel combination or just liquid fuel should be determined; however, fluid of some form should always be a priority for adequate hydration."

Don't forget: In a race or a ride, if for some reason, you only have time to eat or drink, always opt for the drink. The snack will only serve to speed up dehydration as it moves water to your stomach for digestion. "No matter what the preference," McDonald adds, "athletes should stay within the ACSM guidelines of 30 to 60 grams of carbohydrates per hour after the initial hour of exercise."

Whether you are a pro or a recreational

(continues on page 108)

# WHAT THE PROS DRINK

While we may assume professional cyclists gulp down bottle after bottle of highly caloric beverages, the dirty truth is that most of them eschew their sponsored products in favor of good old-fashioned water, sometimes with a pinch of electrolyte powder mixed in to keep things interesting. I thought that most of the pros would have top-secret drink mixes, but I learned that they generally prefer to eat their calories on rides and only occasionally add something other than a basic electrolyte mix to their bottles. There are some exceptions (up to 150 calories in almost every bottle), but for the most part, the pros just prefer the simple stuff—and they like to save their calories for yummier in-ride food.

Here are some fueling tips from the pros:

"I do water if it's pretty basic early-season stuff or if it's not super-hot. Once it becomes really hot and I'm sweating a lot, or if it's midseason and I'm going through a lot of fluids, then I do an electrolyte beverage." —*Ted King, retired pro road racer*

"I drink mainly water, with some electrolytes if it's hot." —*Jeremy Powers, pro cyclocrosser*

"I sweat a lot, so I drink a lot of fluids. I sweat out a lot of electrolytes, and I also didn't grow up eating salt, really. My family just didn't eat salt—we even had unsalted potato chips! I thought that was what potato chips were like. But now I think salt is incredibly strong-tasting. It actually burns my mouth when things are too salty. But as soon as I started mountain biking, I started getting a lot of cramps, and I thought it was from not stretching enough, but I realize now that it was from low sodium. So I use the Clif brand drink mix. They modified their recipe to be a bit less carbohydrate-heavy, and it has more sodium. I drink as much of that as I can, and if it's hot out or I know I haven't been drinking enough, I'll take electrolyte capsules." —*Mo Bruno Roy, retired pro cyclocrosser*

"On the bike, I try to drink a bottle an hour even when it's not hot out. I always have some calories in my bottle—I use straight maltodextrin, which is cheap when you buy it in 50-pound bags. I used to add fruit juice concentrate to give it some flavor, but I don't anymore. I add a bit of salt and put in about 150 calories per bottle, and I bring a baggie of extra powder so I can refill. If you're drinking a bottle an hour with 150 calories, you're doing good with calories without even thinking about it. I also try to keep eating steadily." —*Janel Holcomb, pro road racer*

"I usually just drink water. I'm not a big fan of sports drinks in my bottles because I'd rather just eat my calories. Unless I'm in a race, that is—if I'm doing a mountain bike race or intense intervals, I'll add drink mix." —*Katie Compton, pro cyclocrosser*

"I'll do Clif brand drink mix and shoot for a bottle an hour, generally." —*Georgia Gould, pro mountain biker*

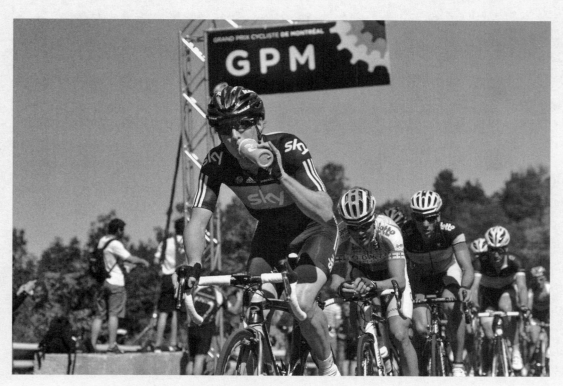

Many pro racers prefer to eat their calories and drink either plain water or an electrolyte solution during races, but it's a highly individual decision.

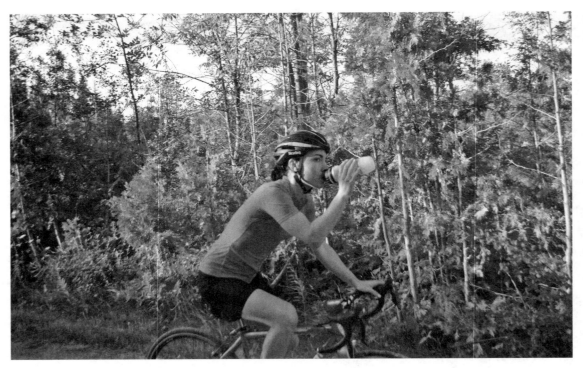

A sports drink can save your ride—especially if you start to feel tired after the first hour.

rider, taking in calories after that first hour on the bike is essential. Carbohydrates are hugely important for mental focus and concentration—there's a reason we want to avoid bonking, not just because it wrecks our chance at a personal best on a hill, but because it's actually dangerous. "The majority of injuries in sports occur when fuel sources are low," cautions Guest. And that's when sports drinks come in handy. "Sports drinks can save a ride—don't be concerned if you didn't eat enough, you can get those simple carbs fast to rescue those muscles that need the fuel," she adds.

## DO I ALWAYS NEED THIS STUFF?

You absolutely do not need to carry on every ride a carbohydrate-dense sports drink. Water is fine for rides under an hour, and if you prefer, you can rely on real food instead of a sports drink for rides over an hour.

"For short and low-intensity rides when it isn't hot out, water is perfectly fine," says nutritionist Jordan Dubé, MS. "Our bodies are able to recoup those electrolytes that we lose as we recover with normal eating and drinking after.

So if you're out for an hour recovery ride, water's going to be okay."

However, when riding in the summer or at a high intensity—and especially if you sweat a lot—you may want to add a pinch of salt or some electrolyte powder to your water. "It's when the temperature or intensity starts to rise that you need to add things into the water," Dubé says. Only in certain situations do rides under an hour require calories.

"In my opinion, while a lot of the really high sugar and carbohydrate drinks may encourage people to drink more, they aren't the best option," she continues. "They're just sugar.

And for most nonprofessional athletes, it's far more sugar than you need."

If you're having trouble leaning out, take a careful look at your scoops of powder and the number of bottles that you consume in a ride—it might be more than you realize, and you might be burning less than you think. "Those people who are religious about sports drinks are sometimes gaining weight or aren't losing the weight that they should through that activity," Dubé says. "I prefer a drink mix that's low-calorie and focuses mainly on electrolyte replenishment. Calories should come from food."

## YOUR FIVE TAKEAWAYS

1. Drink around 16 ounces per hour, but experiment to find what makes you feel and perform the best.

2. If you're riding for more than an hour, make sure you add electrolytes to your water, even if you're not adding calories.

3. You do not need to take in extra calories, especially in drink form, for short rides under an hour (unless it's hot out or at a high intensity).

4. Be aware of the calories in your drinks and factor them into your daily caloric intake.

5. If you are using your drink as your calories, aim for 30 to 60 grams of carbohydrates per hour after the initial hour of exercise, and opt for a blend of sugars rather than simply glucose or fructose.

# CHAPTER ELEVEN

# IN-EXERCISE FOOD

Eating on the bike has never been more—and in some ways, less—complicated. In the past few years, we've seen a major resurgence of real food on rides, including snacking on sandwiches in the peloton, the increased popularity of rice bars, and it's now more acceptable to get that second cookie at the midride coffee stop and bring it with you for your next ride snack. But for every rider who prefers whole foods and hates the newfangled gels, bars, and chews, there's a pro who swears by the processed stuff. So, who's right?

Neither.

Confused? Not to worry—we've got the full explanation. But at the end of the day, the answer is simple. Your perfect ride food is what makes your stomach happy, keeps you from bonking during a ride, and doesn't cause you to pack on pounds like you're training for a sumo wrestling championship. It's a game of trial and error, but there are some basic rules and guidelines to follow.

## PRE-RIDE

Your pre-ride meal may be breakfast, lunch, dinner, or just a snack, but no matter what, it should be eaten with your workout in mind. Eat your pre-ride meal within 1 to 3 hours of training, but for any longer or harder efforts, top off your stores with something small 30 to 45 minutes before hopping on the bike. You can even do this by sipping a sports drink.

"The pre-exercise meal should settle your hunger and help restore carbohydrates to the bloodstream and muscle reserve—the glycogen stores," explains Nanci Guest, MSc, RD, CSCS. Your pre-exercise meal should be the most carbohydrate-heavy of the day with a focus on simple carbs, like rice or oats. In addition to carbohydrates, drink plenty of liquids before your ride: The worst idea is to start a ride when you're already dehydrated—even fasted state training rides should start with you completely hydrated.

Your pre-ride meal is even more important

pre-race, but proper training gives you the chance to play with ratios and see what works best for you. Consider some of your harder interval sessions as a trial race and practice your pre-race meal. Something simple, like oatmeal with maple syrup and raisins, or a rice bowl with almond milk and dried fruit and nuts, is likely going to be your best bet.

Watch out for fiber when consuming a lot of carbohydrates. Some racers have no problem with a pre-race bowl of fruit, but others are sprinting for the restroom before the first corner in a race. "Something like a banana is great, but all fruit doesn't work," Guest adds. "An apple, for example, can cause some digestive upset because it has a lot of fiber. It's great to hold you over between meals, but it's not great for exercise. That fiber is going to aggravate blood supply and potentially cause cramping, nausea, or even fatigue if too much blood is going to your stomach and not your muscles. You want something quick-digesting with just a bit of protein to lower the glycemic index of the simple carb."

A high-fat and high-protein meal takes longer to digest—up to 4 to 5 hours—and can cause you to feel heavy or full, which makes riding uncomfortable. "Avoid high-fat fast foods like hamburgers, french fries, cheese, dishes with heavy oil/cream, and large servings of meat, poultry, or full-fat dairy," Guest says. "Fat is the most important thing to watch out for and avoid immediately before exercise," she adds. "Having

something light like toast with a super thin layer of nut butter and then a glass of skim milk for some protein, that's an ideal pre-training meal."

Don't forget those smaller sources of fat that manage to slip in, often unnoticed. "Adding fat—more than 5 grams—before exercise is going to slow down digestion as well, so avoid that if you're planning to train right away," she explains. "And fat can sneak in—frying eggs in butter, adding a handful of nuts . . . those take hours to get through the system, and you're going to need to let them digest before exercise. Your body won't feel happy."

If there is more time before your ride—closer to 3 hours—feel free to make your pre-ride meal a bit beefier (figuratively or literally). "The longer you have before you exercise, the more food you can safely consume without risking digestive discomfort or nausea," Guest explains.

The amount of calories an athlete should take in depends on a number of factors, including your exercise for that day, your other meals, and your body weight and goals. Simply speaking, that means eating a smaller pre-ride meal if weight loss is your goal versus more food if you're trying to maintain your current weight.

"I think people can save calories by not fueling up so heavily for a training session," she says. "If you're going to work out for an hour, you don't need 600 calories. People worry that they don't have enough fuel for the workout, but I would prefer someone have a smaller snack beforehand and then use a diluted sports drink, maybe only 50 calories over the course of the hour, but keep their energy up and allow them to train more intensely. That's a way to avoid overfueling the system so the calories don't turn into fat. If you add the carbohydrates in small portions to the bloodstream, they'll go where they're really needed and allow the muscles to work out harder." For workouts under an hour, sports drinks should only be consumed when training at a high intensity or in extreme conditions.

Pro road racer Tayler Wiles generally rides in the morning, but she still keeps her breakfast fairly light with a fruit bowl, almond milk, and some nuts. She typically has a small snack closer to the ride and then eats most of her calories on the bike. Her smaller meal strategy is ideal for many riders, especially those who don't have trouble eating on the bike.

"People often overfuel before a workout," Guest says. "You're better off fueling lightly and then fueling throughout the ride, but keeping calories at a minimum. Keep some kind of food on you so you can have it if you need a pick-me-up, but you don't need much to take you far. Just eat as needed, as opposed to trying to over-compensate by having a huge pre-ride breakfast.

"If you're aiming for weight loss," Guest continues, "have a smaller breakfast and add carbs as needed while you're out there so you can better match what you really need." However, don't skimp out on breakfast to the point that you bonk before you even reach the end of the driveway. She explains, "People who are trying to exercise in a low fuel state end up ravenous. If you have an intense training session where you weren't properly fueled, or you did a 3-hour ride on no fuel, it's hard to fight your biology. Afterward, you just binge. You don't feel full until you've completely stuffed yourself."

In order to achieve your performance and nutrition goals, it is essential to fuel in-ride. "To have better control after rides, you need to mitigate getting that extreme hunger by fueling in-ride and pre-ride," she adds. "I believe under any circumstances, if you get to the point where you feel so hungry that bingeing is an issue, that's a problem. It's best to keep your body happy and not do anything extreme. It's around exercise that you want to keep your body happy and well-fueled."

One final thought: It may be tempting to hit the bike while hungry for intense but short rides, but it is important to still top off fuel stores for optimal performance. Be prepared to eat or drink a carbohydrate-rich drink while on the bike to get the most from your workout.

## IN-RIDE

You've had your pre-ride meal, and you're on the bike. Now what? If your ride is longer than an hour, it's time to think about what fuel you need and when you need it. Unfortunately, it's not as simple as eating when you're hungry.

Once you start to feel hungry, you're likely already in danger of bonking, or at least in danger of not being able to put out the power you are capable of.

"As a general rule, in-exercise calories need to be emphasized anytime an athlete plans to exercise or compete for more than 1 hour," says Alexa McDonald, RD, CDN. "In-exercise calories help provide continuous energy, maintain electrolyte balance, and keep blood sugar levels normal to sustain endurance. Carbohydrate intake during exercise has been shown to increase endurance and improve performance."

Most athletes and dietitians agree that refueling after an hour of activity and every 30 minutes thereafter hits the sweet spot for optimal performance. McDonald says, "Athletes should consume 30 to 60 grams of carbohydrates per hour of endurance exercise after the initial hour." Be sure not to overfuel, and only consume the calories needed for your specific ride. For instance, an endurance pace or recovery pace requires less fuel than high-intensity intervals. You don't need to eat and drink calories. Choose the option that works best for you, given the duration and intensity of your ride.

When she isn't racing, pro road racer Janel Holcomb coaches other athletes and notes that while some athletes overfuel, she sees more of a tendency for athletes to underfuel their workouts. "Personally, I think one of the most important aspects of fueling from an athletic perspective is eating enough," she says. "Over the 8 years that I've been a professional, I've seen an enormous number of people who specialize their diets and express their dissatisfaction with their feeling on rides or races. I

## *Janel Holcomb's No-Cook Peanut Butter–Oatmeal Balls*

½ cup peanut butter

4 tablespoons honey, or more as needed

2 cups rolled oats

   Handful of raisins and chocolate chips

Simply combine the ingredients in a mixing bowl (it can get messy), and ball the mixture into tablespoon-size chunks. Add more honey, if needed. For uniform balls, simply spoon the mixture into an ice-cube tray. Place the balls into the fridge for a couple of hours and keep chilled until you are ready to use them. Easy and delicious!

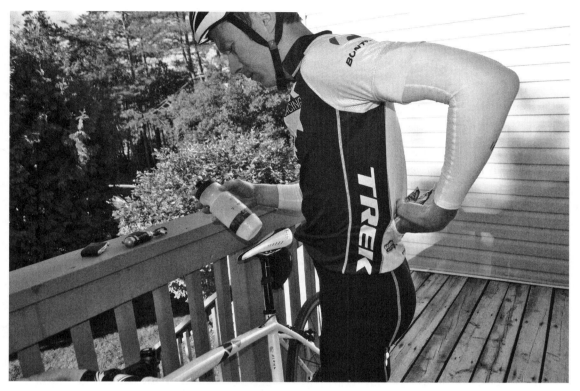

Pre-plan your in-ride food, whether you're making it yourself or just packing gels.

see what they're eating and drinking and how they specialize their diets. But I have a hunch that if they just ate and drank more, they'd feel so good!"

"For me, eating helps me perform," Holcomb continues. "My leanness is an afterthought. What I'm worried about is that what goes in needs to be equal to what goes out in training and racing and what I'm burning when I'm not riding. That's more important—I can't do my job if I'm depriving myself. That's the way that I look at food, and I feel fortunate to do this so I can eat so much food! It's not lost on me that I

get to eat a lot, and I really enjoy it."

That pre-ride meal may have filled up your glycogen stores, but unfortunately, it filled them up equally. When one part of your body reaches exhaustion, you can't transfer unused stores from other areas, so it's imperative to refuel during your long rides. "Even though your shoulders and abs and arms have lots of carbs in them, that's not going to help your quads on a ride, unfortunately," says Guest. "You can't transfer glycogen from one muscle to another. That's why it's better to have a smaller meal pre-ride and fuel during the ride."

"You're only as strong as your weakest link," she continues. "Generally, when you eat, you fill up your muscles with glycogen. But when you start exercising, you only use the glycogen in the muscle that's contracting. So if you're doing a leg strength day at the gym, it's not your biceps or your back or shoulders that are at risk of running out of glycogen, it's your legs. You can't borrow glycogen from other body parts. That's why it's important to keep that in mind when you think about the carb intake before the training session: Only some of them go to the muscles you're using. If you're later in the session, especially an intense one for a particular muscle like your quads while doing sprints, if you don't refuel, you'll fatigue or risk using protein as fuel."

For those of you who have an irrational fear of eating or drinking during your ride because you don't want to waste calories, you're doing more harm than good. Without proper in-ride fuel, your performance will suffer, you risk limiting your recovery, and you'll be more likely to return from your ride ravenous and binge. "Having a sports drink won't make or break your body composition, and drinking it during a workout will only send the carbs where needed, to those depleted muscles—they'll pull it out of the bloodstream," says Guest. "That's why I'm a fan of sports drinks—the muscles that need it will pull it out."

## WHAT TO EAT

While you're riding, carbohydrates—simple ones, particularly—are your friend. It's completely up to you whether you take a whole-foods approach and eat rice cakes or you slurp down some gels, but the macronutrient makeup of your in-ride fuel should be carbohydrate based, for the most part. In longer and more endurance-based rides, you can add more complex foods, even a bit of fat and protein, but simple carbohydrates are king when it comes to high intensity and the best fuel possible for your ride, according to Guest.

Eating while riding isn't going to make you pack on pounds. In fact, if you've had trouble shedding those last few pounds, a properly fueled ride may actually work in your favor and help your body adjust to its best weight.

"The problem is that people think eating nothing means that you burn fat," says Guest. "But there's no exercise that we do that just burns fat. Hours into endurance, you might be burning 60 percent fat, but your body needs carbs." Therefore, make sure your food is carb-heavy to give your body the energy it needs. "Your body can't break down body fat that easily; it's not a simple process. It takes too long. You won't start metabolizing stomach fat to fuel a 3-hour bike ride; it doesn't happen that quickly," she adds.

Just because your body is using carbs doesn't mean you're not burning fat. "You'll still burn fat," Guest explains. "If you eat 100 calories of carbs per hour and you're burning 400 calories per hour, you're going to use fat. You'll use glycogen from muscles, some triglyceride breakdown, and you're going to burn that surplus of calories. Eating or drinking a bit is still going to create a deficit, but that small amount of calories will help you work harder and longer."

Guest breaks down a typical ride, explaining, "For the first hour, you're running on the glycogen stores that are already in your muscles from breakfast and the meals before. By the second, you're running low and you need to top it off, and you rely more and more on added sugars. After a few hours, you're relying entirely on the carbs that you're taking in. If you can't take in what you're burning, you'll slow down. So with a combination of carbs, you can better keep up with the demands of time and intensity because they use different transporters. The shorter a workout is, the more you can rely on glycogen stores. But by that second hour, you need to start taking something in to avoid fatigue."

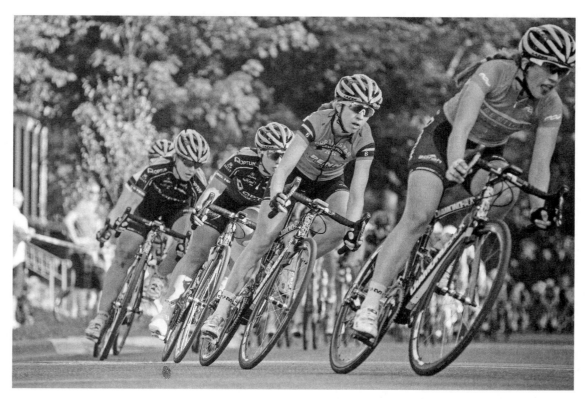

Pro road racer Janel Holcomb swears by gels in races, opting for the simple sugars over whole-foods-based solutions. Her logic? Well, would you want to eat a sandwich while going around that corner?

Go into your ride with a plan and stick to it. If you decide beforehand that you're going to eat a gel or a half an energy bar every 30 minutes, follow through. Don't wait until you hear your stomach growl or start feeling slower or start seeing spots. "You can feel when you're getting hypoglycemic and when you need fuel," says Guest, "but you don't want to risk not having enough fuel. You don't want to ruin your ride. If it turns out at the end of the day that you gained an ounce of fat or that you only lost 4 ounces versus 5, that's not going to make a huge difference. You don't want to wreck your ride."

As a racer already at her goal weight, Holcomb properly fuels her ride to maximize performance and so that she can come home and not panic about recovery. "My approach is that I want my breakfast calories plus my ride calories to be a bit more than what I burn on the ride," she says. "People talk about recovery food, but I don't want to come home and feel like I'm in deficit or that my recovery needs to be within 5 minutes of walking in the door because I'm behind."

Guest warns, "Don't mess with your training" if you are trying to drop a few pounds. "Fuel your training and focus on caloric restriction outside of the training if you want to lose weight."

"I see many athletes eat right at the end of rides, after they have already seen huge performance decline," cycling coach Peter Glassford

adds. "The ride would have probably gone way better, the central nervous system wouldn't have spun up and tried to use proteins to make sugar. . . . If you're going to ride long, just enjoy eating enough in-ride. I think a lot of people try to underfuel in-ride but then end up ravenous at the end and irrational because they're exhausted and their brains have no sugar—so what kind of choices are they making then? Eating enough in-ride may help riders make better choices at the end of the ride." Your performance and recovery will be much stronger if you eat during your ride than if you don't.

## THE CASE FOR WHOLE FOODS

Only eating gels or basic bars on a ride, especially a long, leisurely paced one, can be a huge drag. We ride our bikes because it's fun—so why shouldn't our food be as well? The simple sugars in these packaged items might be what our bodies need for fuel, but the sugars are bad for our teeth and can cause gastrointestinal distress. Besides, gels and sports-specific bars tend to be expensive, and most of us don't have the budget to run through boxes of them every week. So taking a break from traditional processed ride foods in favor of real food isn't just a current trend with serious racers, it's common sense.

"I recommend that clients try making their own bars," says nutritionist Jordan Dubé, MS.

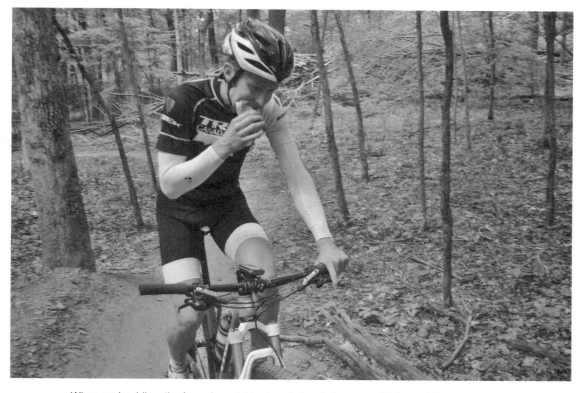

When you're riding, the focus is on taking in calories that you need to keep riding at your best, not on keeping calorie counts low.

"For longer, endurance-paced rides, you can include anything: whole grains, nuts, seeds, dried fruits. I recommend maple syrup or honey to hold them together."

Even simple whole-food staples can properly fuel your ride. Dubé adds, "Almond butter and jelly sandwiches are great, and even easier, bananas are great. They'll get you a lot of the potassium you need on a ride, especially if you're not a good drinker. I tell people to either use something that's easy to whip up right before you ride or something you can make in a big batch and store."

Similarly, Guest suggests dates and peanut butter, saltines with a thin layer of peanut butter and jam, pretzels (for a salty crunch when sweet just isn't appealing), or even simply raisins.

Although Holcomb eats gels during races, she's a fan of whole-foods snacks during regular rides. "In training and racing, it's a bit different. I pack my pockets full with as much real food as I can for training rides," she explains.

She's also not afraid of indulgences in her rides—arguably the best time to sneak in those treats. "I try to make ride stops worthwhile when I do want good food—I stop at pie shops or coffee shops to get something good like pie or hot chocolate. I love real food on the bike, so I'll also make some of it. I'll make little sandwiches—sweet or savory—or my peanut butter–oatmeal balls [see page 116]. I also keep ready-made pie dough in the freezer and make hand-pies—this is where I can make nice savory ones, like scrambled eggs, mashed-up sweet potato, and Parmesan cheese in the dough."

If you just can't quit the gels, it's important to be careful about how you work them into your ride. First, always take the gel with water. "There are two ways taking gels can go wrong," Guest says. "If you take a gel without drinking water, the concentration of sugar in your stomach will draw water in and dehydrate you. You won't absorb it well; it'll sit in your stomach. What you want is a gel mixed with water, which is essentially making a sports drink in your stomach. If it's not diluted, the sugar won't be available for you to use, and you won't get the benefit of the fluid or the carbohydrates. That's true of all solid foods, not just gels—but people seem to make the biggest mistakes with gels."

Second—and this is also true for riders opting for whole foods—be sure to provide your system with plenty of plain water to optimize absorption. "The second mistake people make is washing down a gel with a sports drink, and that's just too concentrated," Guest says. "Your body may still need to pull in water to dilute it, and that can lead to nausea or vomiting as well as dehydration." So when eating your calories, stick to plain water rather than a sports drink.

## THE CASE FOR GELS

If you can't handle whole foods while riding, you may need something that's a bit easier to digest. And in race-specific circumstances, there often isn't time to eat a sandwich or even a bar on the bike. That's where gels and chews come in: They're fast-digesting simple sugars, and while you're off the bike, they're some of the worst kinds of carbs for you. In race situations, they're rocket fuel.

"You see the whole-foods thing becoming a little problematic on the bike," says Glassford. "Off the bike, the whole-foods movement is great, but on the bike, it can cause some issues. You have to look at what you're doing. Whole foods are great, but you're asking a lot of a gut that doesn't have much blood in it in-ride to absorb and process a bunch of coconut oil or almond butter compared to a basic gel. That's the reality, especially when looking at harder riders.

"In a race situation, simple carbs will aid your performance," he adds. "Sometimes, I need to remind the athletes I work with that this whole-foods message is important, but once we are in a high-intensity, performance-oriented workout or race, we need to look to simple carbohydrates to perform at our best. Those simple carbs are not ideal outside of exercise, but I think as we follow this whole-foods trend, we need to be careful we don't jump to an extreme no-carb philosophy and forget years of successful exercise research and practical experience around carbohydrates. I also try to add the perspective that date-based or maple-syrup-based gels or white rice cakes with chocolate and honey are really not any better than maltodextrin powder in terms of nutrient density. It should always come down to 'what is the best fuel for the goal of the day or block of training?'"

Guest adds that gels are designed for intense exercise, and if you're training intensely, it's not the time to worry about sugar. It's time to focus on getting the best fuel for the workout at hand.

Gels are most often used in races, and if you plan to eat gels in competition, make sure to try them out on some training rides first. Glassford explains, "I'm always testing to see what my athletes can stomach and what they will actually eat and drink in race simulations. Some will run drink mix only, some will use fruit, some will use sandwiches, and some will use a combination—but they all find and

practice their strategy based on their individual performances."

There is no need to feel guilty for having a gel in-ride when you eat clean all day. "For most athletes in training, there are only a couple rides each week that need any fueling, so in-ride fueling is a very small contribution to overall nutritional quality," Glassford concludes. Having a gel to fuel your intense ride won't derail your otherwise clean diet.

## HOW THE PROS DO IT

Pro athletes tend to approach nutrition in a similar manner to how they approach their bikes: with an eye toward their sponsors. Remember that just because a pro claims *x* bar and *y* gel are the best things they've ever tried, that doesn't necessarily mean that you should love it, too. If you're not getting paid to eat something, take a step back and think critically about what you put into your body and exactly what you're paying for. Do what is right for your body, your ride, and your nutrition—don't just assume that a pro's choice is the perfect solution for you.

With that in mind, most of the pro racers interviewed for this book opt for gels in race situations, even though they have a serious love of whole foods on the bike.

"I generally don't ride long enough to need food," admits retired pro cyclocrosser Mo Bruno

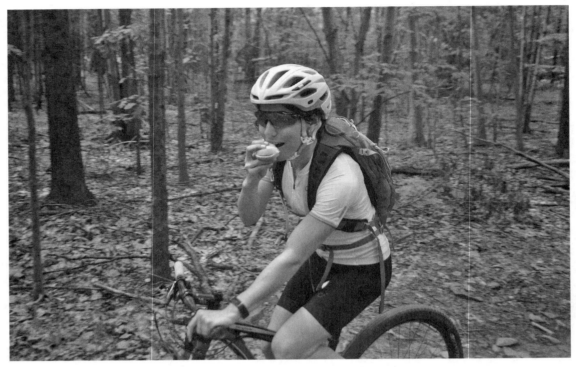

If you're a fan of whole foods, it's easy to make a few staples for rides. Simple sandwiches are a favorite for some, especially when the trails are smooth!

Roy. For a cyclocross racer, that makes perfect sense: Races are between 40 and 50 minutes, and training focuses on short, high-intensity sessions.

When she does fuel in-ride, she limits her consumption. "I have one gel before a race, and I have a two-gel limit regardless of how long a ride is," she explains. "I will bring some Clif Bars with me—their organic ones are three ingredients and are really simple. Or I'll do homemade rice bars or oatmeal-raisin cookies. It's easier to digest real food, and I crave it. Sometimes, I know I need to eat, but nothing in my pocket is interesting to me, so I just need to make something tasty and bring it with me."

Pro mountain biker Georgia Gould prefers to keep her nutrition on the more traditional side for a race, and says, "I'll do a bar or blocks (similar to gel, but in 'gummy' form) every hour or two. I'll use the kid's version of Clif Bars, which are pretty soft and just dried fruit and nuts. If I ride for an hour to 90 minutes, I probably won't eat, but if I'm out for 3 or 4 hours, I'll start eating an hour into the ride and stay on it to give myself steady energy the whole time."

Pro cyclocrosser Katie Compton echoes Bruno Roy's sentiments about eating what makes you happy. "I usually have some healthy bars I can eat. I love Honey Stinger's protein bars and Enduro Bites, which are really good—it's my friend's company and it's all-natural, wheat-free, gluten-free, allergy-free, soy-free. He pretty much made a bar I could eat, and it's awesome." She adds that bars aren't always her go-to, saying, "I'll also put a banana in my pocket, or make my own cookies and put them in my pocket!"

Pro cyclocrosser Jeremy Powers is on the whole-foods bar bandwagon as well and uses training rides as his chance to get creative in the kitchen. "I use a bar or something like that. I make a lot of my own stuff with almond flour, rice, and sweet potatoes, which I mash together to make my own bar with egg and salt. I eat a ton of fruit as well, mainly bananas—but sometimes more than I should!"

Retired pro road racer Ted King arguably puts in the most hours on the bike than any of the other athletes interviewed. "I'm generally drinking a bottle every hour, and if it ends up being a training ride of more than 2 hours, then I generally eat every hour," he explains. "For racing, I'll eat an energy bar, which I'm not too keen on for training, as opposed to in racing. If I'm training, maybe I'll put a bar or two in my pocket, but I'd rather stop at a coffee shop and get a coffee or get a cappuccino or get a cookie or get a muffin. I prefer real food."

King may be slightly biased on his favorite food, but the Vermont native truly does love his whole foods in the form of maple syrup. "I do really think there's something to be said about the real-food movement," he explains. "The same thing that you see in kitchens with the movement toward eating whole foods, real foods—I think the same thing is happening on the bike, too, which is really cool. I'd rather eat an almond rice cake or have UnTapped, my maple syrup single-serve package."

Of all the racers that I spoke with, Wiles is the most anti-gel. "We usually ride after breakfast, and I try to eat every hour: all real food, not bars or gels," she says. "I like to make my ride food: I bake cookies, zucchini bread, banana bread—I like to eat my own food on the bike. I'd rather eat a delicious cookie while riding than a gel! While I'm sometimes not as good about eating every hour, I think it's pretty important to eat consistently in training." She even opts for whole foods during races, which sets her apart from most of the peloton.

## FASTED STATE TRAINING

One of the newest trends in sports nutrition and training is the concept of the fasted state—or glycogen-depleted—ride. This doesn't mean that those underfueled rides that lead to bonking and general crankiness for the rest of the day are good for you. Far from it. Rather, fasted state training is a specific tool, similar to a high-intensity workout with sprint intervals—not something that just happens because you forgot to eat. It's not going to replace your high-intensity rides and shouldn't be used every time you get on the bike.

A fasted state training ride is a shorter endurance or recovery pace ride after a period of fasting—between 10 to 14 hours—so the ride is typically best done in the morning. With a morning training session before breakfast, you've been in a fasted state since dinner the night before.

If you're not a breakfast person, this is where you have an advantage: You can jump-start your training by turning your morning routine into a mini training session in a fasted state (you might even end up wanting breakfast afterward!). "Anyone who wants to improve endurance wants to improve the rate at which they make mitochondria, and that's why training in a fasted state can be really very helpful," Guest adds. Caffeine can add an extra boost to your fasted state session if you just can't get out of bed without it. "You can make that fasted session easier with caffeine," Guest explains.

"One of the most important things that has come out of manipulating carbohydrates in your workout is fasted training," says Guest. "Whether you're high or low carb, there is a benefit to training in a glycogen-depleted state at times." She adds that if you need to eat something in the morning before your workout, you can have pure protein, like a chicken breast. The fasting causes glycogen-depletion, so even if you have a high-protein, no-carb snack, you can still reap the benefits of fasted state training.

In one recent review of the studies surrounding fasted state training, researcher Keith Barr writes that fasted training increases our PGC-1 alpha (peroxisome proliferator-activated receptor gamma, coactivator 1 alpha), an important gene responsible for mitochondrial biogenesis, which leads to the formation of new mitochondria, the "powerhouse of your cells," within muscles.

In order to see gains in our training, we want to increase production of mitochondria in our muscles. One easy way to increase that is through fasted state training. "There's nothing more important to an endurance athlete than increasing the production and activity of mitochondria," explains Guest. "That's the energy production in your muscle cells, and everything else is secondary. Whatever you can do to make more mitochondria means you have the capacity to generate more energy—or adenosine triphosphate (ATP)—which translates into improved speed, power, and endurance. Mitochondria also increase fat oxidation and recall that greater fat use will spare glycogen, and when you're trying to ramp up speed, you'll need that glycogen. Fat won't help you on a hill or while sprinting or anytime you're near lactate or anaerobic threshold."

Barr adds that the point is to do these adaptive sessions, where the muscles are adapting and working to produce more of that mitochondria, in a glycogen-depleted state—the easiest time being before breakfast, after an overnight fast. However, he concludes that these sessions won't be your most impressive. You can expect it to feel significantly worse than a normal session: "It is important to remember that any time training is performed in a fasted or

## FOR WOMEN'S EYES ONLY

For women, hormones can heavily impact exercise, particularly on the days right before and during menstruation. Why? Stacy Sims, MSc, PhD, has spent much of her career trying to find out. If you're a woman whose training is impacted by her cycle, read on.

"Five or 6 days before your period starts is usually when a woman starts to feel off and will want to focus a bit more on hydration and have a bit more carbohydrate, or downplay the amount of protein and fats while exercising so she's able to put out a high intensity and have a bit more cognitive function," Dr. Sims explains. "A really critical thing that people don't talk about is central nervous system fatigue. With elevated progesterone at that time, we have less amino acids circulating, so we tend to have more central nervous system fatigue—that's why women lose their mojo, so to speak."

There is a solution. "Taking in some branched-chain amino acids (BCAAs) before a workout can help with this," Dr. Sims adds. "Now you have an upsurge of amino acids that cross the blood-brain barrier to help delay the onset of that fatigue." BCAAs are found in foods, since they're the building blocks of protein, but taking a BCAA supplement, in either a pill or powder form, is a safe way to incorporate extra amino acids into your diet.

Keep in mind that everyone's body is different and this isn't an across-the-board issue. Some women find that their training isn't as affected during their periods. Each woman has varying hormone levels that react differently, so while you may feel like you're seconds away from bonking 10 minutes into a ride, your friend, who also has her period, may feel fine. If you experience a lot of issues riding during your period, I highly recommend consulting with your doctor or gynecologist.

glycogen-depleted state, the perceived effort will be much higher and performance will decrease."

Think slow, easy, and long. "These adaptive training sessions should be performed at a low absolute intensity for a long time," Barr writes. To get the full benefits, you need to ride for more than 60 minutes, preferably a couple of hours. But don't worry, there are a few ways to trick your body into thinking it's not deprived of glycogen and get through these tough sessions.

Guest adds that not only does fasted state training lead to positive adaptations, it also increases your caloric burn for the day—important for those looking to shed a few pounds—as long as you don't make up those calories the rest of the day. "You want to maximize your total caloric expenditure over a 24-hour period," she says. But it's not the fasting that's creating the fat loss. What you eat the rest of the day (and not bingeing afterward) is key, so it's still a matter of calories in, calories out.

If training in a fasted state is difficult, try tricking your brain a bit. "You can also use a carb mouthwash during fasted training to keep going," Guest explains. "You want to rinse every 10 minutes for about 10 seconds, and amazingly, that tricks the brain into thinking you're drinking carbohydrates. That's great if you want to keep up intensity

but train in a fasted state." However, carb rinses work best for training sessions under an hour, even when you're not at risk of running out of glycogen.

Alternatively, Guest adds, you can use caffeine—so enjoy that cup of coffee (or caffeine tablets or gels) before you ride—to rescue high intensity in a fasted state. "We consistently see up to a 3 percent benefit with caffeine, which is huge," she says. So, for example, a 40-kilometer cycling time trial without caffeine could take you 55:00 minutes, while with caffeine, that 3 percent improvement could get you down to 53:21. That's a big shift!

It is important to avoid antioxidants, especially in supplement form, during fasted state training. "Make sure you don't have too many antioxidants in pill form," says Guest. "More antioxidants interfere with low-grade free radical production. Athletes are producing more free radicals—by default they're at a higher level because they're going through a higher level of metabolism during exercise. So you'd think they'd need more antioxidants; however, it was shown those free radicals are part of the stimulation that will increase the mitochondria. So if you're interfering and neutralizing those free radicals, your body isn't adapting. That's where it comes back to diet and these high-dose supplements being problematic."

While fasted state training has its benefits,

| | DO IT WHEN . . . | HOW OFTEN | EFFECT |
|---|---|---|---|
| **Fasted state or glycogen-depleted state training** | You've fasted overnight or 2nd ride w/out refuel from 1st ride to increase your mitochondria | 2–3 times per week | Stimulate the PGC-1 alpha gene expression and increase mitochondria |
| **Caffeine before/ during training** | When you want a boost in your training, helps rescue a good session fasted and also nonfasted | 2–3 times per week (and make sure to test if you want to do pre-race) | Improve power, energy and focus; increase your pain threshold; and decrease your perceived effort levels |
| **30–60 g of carbohydrate per hour after 1st hour, up to 80 g per hour after 4th hour** | You want your best training ride | Anytime | Proper fueling leads to fast legs—important in interval training and on long rides |
| **No antioxidants in your system** | You've fasted overnight and didn't have anything high in antioxidants in the 12 hours before | When training in a fasted state | Stimulate the PGC-1 alpha gene expression and increase mitochondria |

it is not an excuse to skip breakfast, and it definitely shouldn't be done every day. "You don't want to always train in a fasted state because you may end up in gluconeogenesis—where the body starts breaking down protein to use as fuel. Remember, fat can only provide a small amount to the fuel mix, and guess where this protein comes from? That's right, from your muscles," says Guest. "If you don't like eating in the morning, sip on diluted fruit juice (a 1:1 ratio) or sports drink before and during exercise just to protect that protein and to get your blood sugars up. It's not heavy so you won't have to battle for the blood supply trying to digest it.

"You'll have a better training session if you're properly fueled, and that's why you can't train in a fasted state all the time. The constant influx of small amounts of carbs into your bloodstream is protein-sparing and makes the brain and muscles just happy enough to let you perform at a decent intensity," says Guest. "But fasted state training is something that has been shown to help with body-fat loss and that stimulation of the PGC-1 alpha, which is responsible for mitochondrial biogenesis. And the more mitochondria you have, the more aerobic capacity you have."

Other than as a way to boost your caloric deficit for the day, don't expect training while hungry to help you shed pounds at a faster rate. In a recent study of 20 women by fitness expert Brad Schoenfeld, PhD, CSCS, there was no change in body mass after fasted exercising versus unfasted states. So if you're looking to lose a few pounds, avoiding a pre-ride snack may not be the best way to do it.

To that end, there are plenty of times fasted state training isn't the answer, says Guest. "There are times you want to do training in a fasted state, but if you're looking to get more fitness and have more intensity in your training session, you don't want to mess with that fine line of having enough fuel. If you don't have enough, you risk starting to use muscle proteins, and that's not a clean-burning fuel. Furthermore, you won't improve fitness if you can't train at those high intensities. High-intensity training needs fuel and is necessary to improve your aerobic and anaerobic capacity. Increasing your lactate threshold—the point in exercise where lactic acid starts to build up in the bloodstream—is the most important goal to increase race pace for endurance athletes."

If you start to feel sore on a regular basis, decrease the times per week that you train in a fasted state. Guest cautions: "Over time, someone doing that a lot will have more soreness, more injuries, and a compromised immune system. When you train in that carb-depleted state, your body is stressed and releases cortisol. Cortisol stimulates gluconeogenesis, and cortisol's weakening effects on the immune response have also been well documented. But we do need cortisol—it also stifles inflammation due to the inhibition of histamine secretion. Cortisol's ability to prevent an adequate immune response can render individuals suffering from chronic stress—psychological or through too many low-fuel or fasted rides—highly vulnerable to infection or slowed recovery from training. Over time, that's why we see athletes susceptible to respiratory infections, and that's partially because they're not taking in enough fuel. Consuming enough carbohydrates is the most ideal to suppress cortisol from being released."

# YOUR FIVE TAKEAWAYS

1. Take in simple carbs in the form of gels or whole foods for rides more than 1 hour.

2. After your first hour of riding, consume 30 to 60 grams of carbohydrates hourly. Aim for the higher end during intense sessions and even up to 80 grams per hour in the fourth or fifth hour of a superlong ride. This is not associated with body weight!

3. Your ride isn't the time to start a diet: Fuel for the way you want to ride.

4. Try different in-ride foods: Experiment with whole foods and gels to find out what works the best for you. You may need different foods for racing versus training rides.

5. If you're looking for a new way to train, consider fasted state training by riding on an empty stomach (after 10 to 14 hours of fasting, usually ideal before breakfast), but remember to keep the intensity low and don't mistake fasted state training for a bonked ride.

# CHAPTER TWELVE

# IN-RACE FOOD

R ace day can be stressful no matter how prepared you are. Like many riders, you may wake up feeling slightly nauseated, or you may require an extra trip or two to the porta-potty before the race start. Unfortunately, this is always the case for many of us, but the good news is that there are ways to improve the situation so you can start the race properly fueled and hydrated, without butterflies in your stomach.

Endurance athletes (those of you doing any exercise more than 1 hour) deal with two problems: pre-race fueling and in-race food and hydration. Having an in-race nutrition plan before the start of an event can mean the difference between winning and losing, or even finishing. When I competed in an Ironman (2.4-mile swim, 112-mile bike ride, followed by a 26.2-mile run)—sorry to out myself as a triathlete—I was young and inexperienced and I didn't know the significance of having a fuel plan. The result? I skipped breakfast because my stomach was in knots as I waited for the swim to begin. Then, I ate four gels and drank four bottles of water with no added electrolytes on the 112-mile bike ride. By mile 3 of the run, my legs cramped, and I was bonking. No matter how much I tried to eat, my body rebelled because it was in such shock already. Dry-heaving for the last 10 miles, I finished the race much slower than I'd hoped. My most vivid memory of that night was sitting in the shower of my hotel room, crying, and sipping vegetable broth from a can.

Oh, the glamorous lives of racers.

It's actually not that hard to avoid the dreaded bonk. It just takes some common sense and a willingness to develop a fueling plan and to stick with it.

## YOUR PRE-RACE MEAL

Similar to your pre-ride meal, focus on replenishing glycogen stores a couple of hours before your race, and then top off your tank closer to the starting time. Pre-race meals should focus primarily on carbohydrates, particularly mild ones.

(continues on page 134)

# TUMMY TROUBLE

Plenty of us experience a bit of stomach distress in the form of butterflies or an urgent trip to the restroom once or twice (or 10 times) pre-race. But there are also a lot of us who have stomach complaints almost on a daily basis. Stress, posture, personal food sensitivities, and less-than-helpful diagnoses like irritable bowel syndrome can make riding seem a lot more like work than fun.

Balancing your gut's microbial makeup can be tough, especially when training a lot, but it's possible to cut down on some of the particularly painful symptoms. First, don't rely on painkillers for sore muscles. They risk masking symptoms or significant injuries and can hurt your digestive system overall. Studies have shown that taking ibuprofen prior to a ride can cause leakage in the small intestine, and constant usage may lead to compromised intestines. Sounds great, doesn't it?

Studies have shown that 30 to 50 percent of athletes complain of gastrointestinal (GI) distress during exercise, according to a recent review by Erick Prado de Oliveira at the Federal University of Uberlândia. Often the distress happens when exercising at high intensities, as opposed to on recovery days, which explains why stomach issues may be exacerbated in race situations.

Stomach issues present themselves in any number of ways, including cramping, diarrhea, nausea, constipation, and bloating. Unfortunately, there's such individual variation that it's impossible to pinpoint one specific symptom, but there are a few ways to identify individual causes and work to improve stomach issues.

Posture while riding relates to certain stomach issues—you might be in the ideal aerodynamic position, but breathing heavily while hunched over can lead to upper gastrointestinal symptoms, explains Oliveira, and they may be more common "possibly due to increased pressure on the abdomen as a result of the cycling position." Additionally, he notes, swallowing air while breathing heavily and drinking from water bottles (more air bubbles) can also add to stomach troubles.

The good news is that your body will adapt as you spend more time in the saddle.

Breaking up your carbohydrate sources can also help avoid stomach issues. Too much of one sugar—glucose or fructose, for example—can lead to stomach distress, so search for gels and drinks with multiple sources. Oliveira recommends shifting away from foods that are high in fructose if you experience severe stomach cramps and pain on the bike.

There are several key ways to keep stomach problems at bay during training. First, as we've already learned, avoid eating large quantities of high-fiber foods before exercise. Normally, this means not eating them within 2 to 4 hours of training, but for bigger competitions, avoid high-fiber foods for a full day beforehand. That said, a high-fiber diet on noncompetitive days, Oliveira notes, is good for athletes, as the fiber will help regulate your bowel movements.

Unfortunately, women run a higher risk of GI distress in exercise. "A woman may not do as well with maltodextrin or fructose," says Stacy Sims, MSc, PhD. "In choosing things to eat on the bike, a woman should avoid stuff like dried fruit to avoid fructose and fiber," she explains. "When you have that in the intestine, it exerts a strong pressure, and the body's response is to dilute it with water, which can lead to GI distress and dehydration. More women have GI distress and hyponatremia [too much water, too little electrolytes], which can be brought back to what she's eating."

Hydration is also key in preventing stomach distress. As our bodies become dehydrated, any existing stomach problems become even more exacerbated. Staying hydrated while ingesting food is also important in order to avoid your stomach leaching water from elsewhere in the body to break down what it just took in. To avoid this, drink enough water on the bike (and learn how to drink while riding), but don't forget about hydrating off the bike throughout the day. Hydration is especially important with pre-ride meals.

Lastly, as cycling coach Peter Glassford notes, it's crucial to practice race-day nutrition to avoid stomach upset. Knowing what foods and drinks trigger stomach pain—or more important, knowing which won't hurt your stomach—can go a long way toward having a positive race-day outcome.

"In general, eating more mild foods for race day is key," says nutritionist Jordan Dubé, MS, "and eat familiar foods!" This isn't the time to try out that awesome-looking breakfast burrito that the food truck vendor is selling by the start line. This is when you stick to what you know.

Dubé reiterates that fiber pre-race is rough on the system: "Nothing with too much fiber. Fiber is great, but on race day, fiber is not your friend."

Practice is key as well. You practice your racing with hard intervals, group rides, and skills sessions, so practicing how you fuel is simply another piece of the puzzle. "Just like not all training methods work for all people, not all meal plans work for all people," Dubé says. "So practicing a race-day eating plan on a day you have a hard training effort is essential. Knowing that your body can tolerate certain foods on race day is important to practice. Never try new foods at a race! Know what your body is comfortable with before you get there."

Race days can be stressful for even the most prepared racer, but you can help your day run smoothly by having your nutrition pre-packed. Don't count on a race to have a vendor serving the exact sports drink that you want. I've even been to races that ran out of water bottles, and without any potable water on-site, I raced with empty bottles and hadn't had a sip for nearly an hour pre-race. Needless to say, they weren't my best performances.

To avoid a similar race-day crisis, be pre-pared and pack all of the supplies, food, and drinks you'll need to support your ride, Dubé says. "You need to bring food you know (and know everything that's in it). Making recipes you're familiar with and taking them with you to races can eliminate the problems you might have. If you're stopping at a doughnut shop or a diner on the way to the race or eating from a food truck at the race, how can you expect to feel good?"

Consume your pre-race meal well before the start time so you can make an extra trip to the restroom, if needed—3 hours is usually a good window, but if you have a nervous stomach, test out eating a bit earlier, even 4 or 5 hours earlier. However, the farther from your race start time that you eat your main meal, the more likely you'll need to sip on a watered-down sports drink to keep your glycogen stores steady. Then, within 30 to 45 minutes of your race, try to take in around 100 calories of simple carbohydrates. This is where gels, simple bars, and sports drinks come in handy. Again, practice this routine before a workout to make sure it works for you.

## IN-RACE FOOD

One of the most important things to remember is to stick with what you know on race day, and keep it simple. It is not the time to test out a cool new gel pack or eat the unknown bar that came with your race number and free T-shirt.

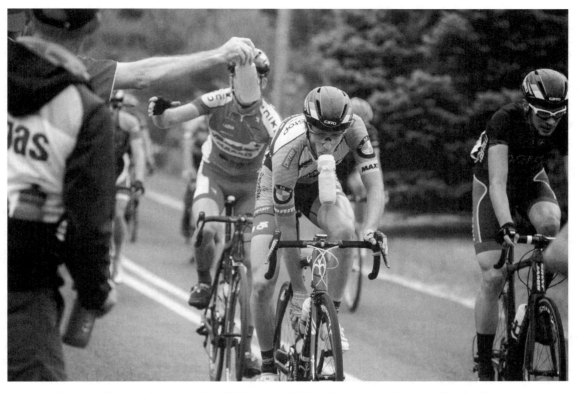

Having a plan to make sure you're drinking enough is key. In pro races, there are often feed zones, so riders can restock on extremely long courses.

Practice your race-day eating the same way that cyclocrossers practice barriers: It's a skill, just like bunny hopping or accelerating off of the start line. Races are often won and lost as a result of good or bad in-ride food choices, and even the pros are susceptible to mistakes. Alberto Contador crashed out of the Tour de France in 2014 because he went for a gel in his pocket and ended up on the ground. If even the best riders in the world can mess up a feed, you can bet it's worth your time to practice the skill of in-race eating.

"For at least one or two workouts in your week, you're going to want to do a 'race simulation' with nutrition," says cycling coach Peter Glassford. "Practice pulling bars or gels out of your pockets, practice drinking while pedaling. It's great for improving skills and testing tolerances—you can see what works ideally for your body."

Practicing your race-day eating is essential to prepare your stomach and learn what works best for you. If you typically eat whole foods on your rides but prefer something simple like a

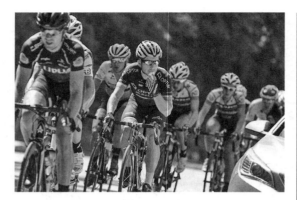

It's not always easy to eat during a race, especially one where you're racing in the peloton. Try going on group rides and eating what you normally would in a race to get comfortable with eating while staying in a pack.

gel—as many of the pros do—in a race, you should occasionally eat a gel during training rides so it doesn't come as a shock to your system on race day.

It's hard to eat, and certainly hard to chew-swallow-repeat, in high-intensity race situations, which is why most of the racers I've interviewed prefer to take their calories in gel or drink form during a race. Think about it: A gel will never be a choking hazard but a muffin might.

Pro road racer Janel Holcomb loves to eat whole foods during training, but she would never consider them for racing. "For racing, the main difference is that instead of having calories in both bottles, I have one bottle that's just water," she says. "That's because in racing, I'll inevitably eat gels, and you need to wash those down with water. When the intensity goes up and the racing is busy, you can't sit back and have a turkey-and-cheese sandwich! You're

just working too hard to be able to do that. So when the intensity goes up, I try to eat more food earlier so that when it gets crazy, I'm not worried."

Pro road racer Tayler Wiles is on the opposite side of the in-race fueling spectrum. "I never eat gels anymore, even in races," she says. "Our soigneurs make us these delicious paninis or little waffles with peanut butter or Nutella. If I eat a gel anymore, it makes me sick!" She does admit though, "If I really, really need something in the last 30 minutes of a race, I'll eat a gummy block—it's filled with sugar but it is pretty easy on the stomach and gives quick energy."

## RACE TRAVEL

One of the biggest things a racer can do to improve their race-day routine is to simply not stress out. Don't worry if your morning meal wasn't exactly what you wanted or you were running late getting to the start: Stressing out is only going to tie your stomach in knots and make your race even harder.

Pre-race stress can negatively impact your performance, especially if the race isn't close to home. You can mitigate those circumstances the best that you can, but staying calm and looking at your nutrition in the big picture is the easiest way to have your best race.

There are simple ways to avoid the added stress from traveling with these tips from Holcomb. "Time zones mess with your internal clock and system a lot, which can be a huge pain. I'm super-aware of how well-hydrated I am before, during, and after travel. I try to drink a lot and that helps," she continues. "But I also try to eat a lot of vegetables and fruit, especially on long flights. I think when I do that, it helps my system stay regular and helps me feel better about being stuck on a plane."

Retired pro road racer Ted King adds, "I used to be a lot more picky about nutrition on the road, but then I realized that's a huge added stress when you're racing, and you're already stressed about a bunch of things. So I've tried to be more flexible. For long flights, I try to take a lot of food with me because relying on airplane food is tough. But I try to stay open-minded because so often, we don't have control over what we're going to eat, and I think if you get too crazy about it, it adds too much stress."

In summary, prepare for both local races and ones that you travel to as best as you can by packing all of the food, drinks, and supplies that you need. Don't worry if something does not go exactly as planned. Adding stress to the equation will only make matters worse.

## YOUR FIVE TAKEAWAYS

1. Your pre-race meal should be carbohydrate-heavy and eaten about 3 hours before competition.

2. Top off glycogen stores 30 to 45 minutes pre-race with around 100 calories of simple carbs, like a gel or sports drink.

3. Practice your in-race nutrition during training rides. Try out what you will eat, when you will eat it, and your fueling technique.

4. Stick to simple carbohydrates during your race for optimal fast-burning fuel. Gels are typically preferred for racing, but experiment to determine what works best for you.

5. Stay calm. Race morning won't always be perfect. Travel can wreak havoc on your nutrition, but letting stress get to you only makes the situation worse.

# CHAPTER THIRTEEN

# POST-RIDE FOOD

Post-ride eating causes one of two emotions: excitement or panic. Some people are thrilled to be done with the ride and are ready to celebrate the accomplishment with a well-earned snack. Others panic as soon as they walk in the door, terrified that the window to refill glycogen stores and take in muscle-repairing protein is seconds away from slamming shut forever.

Or maybe, we're just hungry.

Whatever the case, remember that an immediate post-ride meal is important, but it's not as important as you likely think. If you've fueled your ride adequately, you shouldn't walk in the door feeling like a ravenous wolf.

Pro road racer Janel Holcomb is a huge proponent of simply eating enough on rides to avoid needing an immediate recovery meal. "I want to be ahead by the time I walk in the door, so I don't have to worry as much about making myself a shake or something," she says. "I walk in the door, and I can have whatever I want. If I'm hungry, I eat. If not, I jump in the shower and then I eat. I'd rather be happy and not bonking on the bike than be behind on calories and need to worry about it when I get back."

Holcomb is right by making sure she walks in the door still feeling satisfied from her in-ride food so that she doesn't end up pigging out on junk food because she's in a sugar-crashed state. Recovery is important, that much is definite. "Athletes need to pay attention to the three R's after exercise," Nanci Guest, MSc, RD, CSCS. "Rehydrate, replenish muscle glycogen, and repair damaged proteins. Effective adaptation to training will occur only if all three R's are attended to.

"You need to replenish glycogen stores if you're training again that day," says Guest. "But if you have 24 hours, that's plenty of time if you're getting enough total carbs throughout the day. And if you're not training to any great extent for 2 days, that's even more recovery time. Where immediate recovery becomes an issue is for people training twice a day, something like a ride in the morning and weights in the afternoon. So you need the glycogen so you're ready for your weight set," she adds.

The three key ingredients to recovery, as Guest mentions, are fluids, to rehydrate; carbohydrates, to replenish glycogen stores; and protein, to start repairing and adapting muscles. "When I have athletes with training sessions close together, I want them to have quick-absorbing carbs right away," she explains. "Repairs won't be made right between sessions, but then you want to have a protein-rich meal at night to make sure you repair and do that building overnight. You need to think every day about your food being part of your recovery for the next training session, unless you're only training every 4 days."

For optimal recovery during hard training blocks, the rules about eating right before bed change—but don't think this is an excuse to eat dessert late at night. Guest says that one key to ideal recovery and adaptation is a nightly dose of protein, around an hour before hitting the sheets. Contrary to popular belief, having calories right before bed won't immediately turn to fat, unless you're over the amount of calories you needed for the day. "We want to minimize how long we go without protein," Guest explains, "and this helps with our training and recovery."

"Anyone training regularly should have a good dose of protein before bed," she says, "even when aiming for fat loss or planning fasted state training the next morning since fasted state training is mainly focusing on not having carbohydrates." Even a small dose of protein is preferable to nothing, so don't panic if you can't get that full 20 grams in right before bed.

Combining the protein with a bit of fat, like Greek yogurt, will slow down absorption so it releases slower while you sleep—then when you wake up, you've only gone a few hours without protein. This can be a huge benefit for athletes ramping up their training—even those ramping up training for fat loss. "You want to be able to train hard the next day," Guest says. "This ensures that you can recover and maintain those high-intensity sessions day after day and week after week. Whether your goal is fat loss or improved performance, you're only as good as how well you have recovered. If you don't recover properly and are overtrained, you may need to take a lot more time off, which sabotages your ability to improve performance or lose weight, because you won't have that higher-calorie burn from high-intensity sessions."

Proper recovery is key to improved overall performance. You want your post-ride meal to contain all of the nutrients you need: primarily protein, carbohydrates, and electrolytes.

Pro road racer Tayler Wiles shares her (and

## THE SMOOTHIE ALWAYS WINS

Some athletes prefer to sit down to a full meal three times a day plus a solid snack before or after training, but that just isn't realistic for most of us. What is easy for the average cyclist are leftovers, as we discussed in the lunch and dinner chapters, and smoothies. We're not talking about store-bought junk that largely features apple juice. We're talking about ones that you blend yourself. With a decent blender, you can easily make a smoothie to sneak in a few extra servings of vegetables, tons of fiber with fruits and leafy greens, and a solid 20-gram dose of protein (the convenience of whey protein powder or Greek yogurt is perfect here!). It's a fast-delivery system, and you can tailor your smoothie to fit your caloric and macronutrient needs. There are tons of recipes out there, but the best thing to do is just start experimenting.

A lot of the pros like to incorporate shredded beets in their smoothies for some sweetness and a kick of vitamins. Spinach is also popular and easy to break down. Frozen berries provide a good backdrop for the whey protein powder, and extras like cucumbers are great for adding more liquid and fiber, with a refreshing coolness. If you want more calories because you're subbing a smoothie for a meal, include specific ingredients based on your caloric needs. For more protein calories, add a base of Greek yogurt or whey protein powder; for more carb calories, add bananas or juice; if you want to add fat calories, add flaxseed oil; and if you're trying to keep calories low, water and ice are great.

A simple smoothie recipe is one scoop of chocolate whey protein powder, a cup of frozen blueberries, and a teaspoon of chia seeds or flaxseed oil. Put the ingredients in a blender with about 2 cups of water or ice. Blend and enjoy!

As the seasons change, switch up your smoothie routine with new nutrients and flavors: in the fall and winter, I love pumpkin puree with a bit of cinnamon, nutmeg, and vanilla whey protein powder blended together with ice for a milk-shake-*esque* treat.

This is a travel-friendly, delicious, and sneaky way to cram in post-ride nutrition even when you need to get on with your day! Experiment with various ingredients to find a combination that works best for you.

fellow pro road racing riding partner, Olivia's) post-ride recovery plan. "When we get back, we always do a recovery smoothie within 30 minutes of riding, and within 2 hours, we eat a real meal. Sometimes, we eat just left-overs from the night before, and sometimes, we do eggs with rice cakes and avocado and some kind of veggie." By having a smoothie right away, Wiles manages to get in the protein she needs and quell hunger pangs until she can clean up, relax, and prepare her next meal.

While recovery is important after long, hard rides, it's equally important to ask yourself if you really need to recover. How intense was your ride? If you did an hour of super-easy rid-ing, you don't need a protein shake at the end of it—you can easily wait an hour and have a real meal with whole foods.

The recovery meal is just that: recovery. It's not a reward or an indulgence. A cupcake isn't recovery, unfortunately. If you stop thinking of recovery meals as the reward to a ride well done, it may help you be more honest about what you actually need. I personally prefer to keep my recovery meal simple and something I'm not overly excited about: a quick smoothie with some frozen fruit and whey protein pow-der. It's tasty, yes, but I don't dream about drinking it. Treating your recovery meal like the last leg of a workout should help keep you from overindulging.

"People tend to reward themselves too much when they didn't work out too hard," says Guest. "For example, look at someone who left the house at 8:00 a.m., got ready to ride, pumped up tires, checked his chain, packed up his saddlebag, then rolled out of the driveway. He meets a friend to grab a cof-fee before the ride and then hits the road with his buddy, stops to take some pictures, maybe has another coffee. He gets lost, has to stop to check maps, and he hits a lot of stoplights coming back into town. By the time he gets back, it's 12:30 p.m., and he thinks, 'I did a $4\frac{1}{2}$-hour ride.' But you have to stop and think, 'How much time did I actually spend riding?'"

Once you do the math, clearly a high-calorie recovery meal isn't necessary in this case. "It's easy to think $4\frac{1}{2}$ hours should mean you can eat whatever you want. People reward them-selves for lower-intensity workouts, but that's what you need to be careful about," Guest cautions. "If you've been out for 5 hours, you feel hungry even if you didn't ride the whole time, and you feel more inclined to reward yourself because you've been exercising. That's when people don't see their desired results: They overestimate calories burned. Four hours might mean over 1,500 calories burned, but if you only really rode for two of them, that's a lot less."

Recovery is not as urgent as once thought. Eating immediately after a ride gets refueling out of the way and can save you from bingeing later in the day. But if you don't have your recovery meal within 30 minutes, don't panic: Your muscles aren't at risk. And remember, don't eat if you're not hungry, unless the refueling is critical for a second training session that day.

# YOUR FIVE TAKEAWAYS

1. Fuel your ride properly so you're not starving when you get home.

2. The recovery window is longer than you think, but eating right away can reduce the risk of bingeing later.

3. A recovery meal should consist of protein and carbohydrates. Don't forget to rehydrate.

4. Every ride doesn't warrant a recovery meal: Be sensible. Your nutrition should match your performance.

5. On heavy training days, try to get in an extra dose of protein just before going to bed to promote muscle repair and adaptation.

# PART FOUR

---

# YOUR BODY

A s cyclists, part of what makes us fast is being lean. Ideally, you want muscle without bulk, and as little extra body fat as possible. Cyclists come in all shapes and sizes, but across the board, the winners are lean.

If you're reading this book, the odds are good that in addition to learning how to fuel your ride to achieve optimal performance, either you're working to maintain your weight or you have a bit of excess that you'd like to trim—most of us do! Unfortunately, sometimes just putting in long or hard hours on the bike won't cut it when it comes to dropping those last few pounds.

That's why the last part of this book is dedicated to your body and weight loss: not the kind where you'll be skinny in 3 weeks, or a 10-day miracle diet, but rather, real results that may take a while to achieve, but once you do, will last. The process is not even painful! Weight loss is all about small changes to your diet. Now that you've read the last few chapters, you already have a good idea of what those changes are: Cut out processed foods, unnecessary fats, and low-quality carbohydrates and consume more vegetables and lean protein.

Weight loss is a pretty simple equation of calories in and calories out. Sure, genetics may dictate that some people burn certain macronutrients better than others, and a genetic test (see Appendix: Testing on page 191) can provide you with the information to shift your macronutrient breakdown into the optimal fat-burning mode. But for the rest of us, there are plenty of simple weight-loss strategies that will work no matter what your DNA may be.

The basic rules are simple. Calculate calories in and calories out so you're burning slightly more than you're eating. You can sneak in extra caloric savings in the meals that aren't directly around your ride. But above all, try to keep your cycling at its peak level, and remember that when you're on the bike, you're not thinking about weight loss, you're focusing on optimal nutrition.

In the following chapters, we will address not only weight loss but also other factors such as stress, supplements, and immunity and how they can impact your nutrition and performance.

# CHAPTER FOURTEEN

# WEIGHT LOSS

How do you fuel for an active lifestyle while eating little enough to shed pounds? Pro racers obviously manage to balance being light enough to get up hills fast without sacrificing any of their power to do so. But for those of us who aren't genetically gifted or have other focuses outside of cycling, it may be a bit harder to keep that extra weight off.

The first step is knowing what you want. As a cyclist, the number on the scale isn't the only number you should consider, and if you see that number drop and your power drops at the same time, shedding weight is actually hurting your cycling. This book is about being the best cyclist that you can be, so focus on keeping your power up while working toward your goal weight. Keep your goals fluid and reassess throughout the process. You may discover that a weight slightly above—or below—what you thought was your goal weight is where you feel the best and have the most impressive power output.

"It's all about finding that balance between being under- and overfueled," says cycling coach Peter Glassford. "On a given day, it helps to consider the amount and type of fuel your daily workout needs, based on norms or your past experience—while watching your power-to-weight ratio and making sure that your workout quality is progressing. That will guide your nutrition over the long term. Unfortunately, as an athlete, you can't just rely on the scale. You need to use other metrics: Know your 20-minute threshold power, or if you don't train with power, know how fast you climb a certain hill near home. That way, as you slowly and steadily drop weight, you can see if your numbers or times are improving or if they're deteriorating, and you can reevaluate your goals, as needed. And if you know you're close to your goal size, you may want to focus less on the scale and more on how clothes fit, and how you look in a mirror."

"It's part of reading your body," explains retired pro road racer Ted King. "So I really don't like standing on the scale, but you understand when your pants are looser or tighter. You understand when you see an extra rib if you're looking in a mirror. It's a more subjective stance on nutrition and fitness and health and weight rather than obsessing about it."

The occasional weigh-in is great—and if you have a lot of weight to lose to hit your goal, it can be a big motivating factor in your weight-loss success—but what's really important for a cyclist is a more overall focus on health. Your true body-fat percentage is actually the best measure for weight loss. That's the number you want to lower, not necessarily your overall weight.

Be careful not to use one of those easy online calculations. Body mass index (BMI) calculators are intended for the general public, and that calculation assumes that most of your muscle is actually fat. As athletes, we have a much higher percentage of muscle mass, so BMI calculators are actually useless for an athletic body type. For example, according to BMI scales, most bodybuilders are considered morbidly obese, when in actuality they have under 5 percent body fat. "When talking about athletes, you never want to use BMI," says Nanci Guest, MSc, RD, CSCS. "It's the one group you shouldn't use it for, because it's so inaccurate for them. Nearly every athlete is overweight according to BMI, unless you're incredibly slim and have almost no extra muscle. I love the Bod Pod, or even underwater weighing. But

calipers or a bioimpedance device or scale are probably the most practical."

So what should you be aiming for? According to Stacy Sims, MSc, PhD, essential fat—fat we need to survive—is 4 percent for men and 12 percent for women. But you should aim for something more realistic. Men in peak cycling condition should aim for no lower than 7 or 8 percent, while women should strive for at least 15 to 17 percent for ideal fitness. Dr. Sims says, "Those numbers, though, are hugely individual from person to person. There are lean, healthy people with numbers 10 percent higher than that essential number. If you're only a few points off of those 'optimal numbers,' don't panic. Someone's best performance may not come from the low numbers."

Another important question to ask yourself before you continue with this chapter is: Do you really need to focus on weight loss? You may see some improvements in your riding by just changing the way you eat. If you haven't been adhering to a clean, nutrient-dense diet with appropriate amounts of protein, then consider adapting to a whole-foods-focused diet with appropriately fueled rides before worrying about counting calories.

Similarly, are there any low-hanging fruits you can tackle to improve your cycling before restricting your diet to drop pounds? Maybe you can work on your technical skills for an extra hour a week or add more hill repeats to

# THE CASE FOR WEIGHING IN

Whether you struggle with weight or not, stepping on the scale once a week can be your biggest defense against extra poundage sneaking on. If you don't have a bioimpedance scale (which can estimate body fat), a regular bathroom scale is better than nothing.

A recent study in Finland by Elina Helander, a senior scientist at the Arctic Centre at the University of Lapland, showed a correlation between weighing in and weight control. Subjects who weighed in at least once a week were more likely to lose weight or maintain their current weight, while those who took weeks away from the scale found the weight they'd lost creeping back.

Another study by Meghan Butryn, PhD, research assistant professor in the department of psychology at Drexel University, looked at more than 4,000 dieters, and it showed the importance of weighing yourself regularly. The study concluded that "maintaining or increasing self-weighing frequency . . . was associated with less weight regain." So even once you've dropped the pounds, it's essential to check in on a regular basis to keep them off.

If you're truly scale-adverse (and I don't blame you), try using a measuring tape around your waist and thighs once a week—it provides a great indication of whether you're dropping fat and replacing it with muscle. Use this technique in combination with the scale (if you can) for a fuller picture of your body composition.

Although weekly weigh-ins are not the most fun thing in the world, they're an easy way to keep motivated and on task because they lessen the chance that you'll let your training or diet slip. Weekly weigh-ins are also a good indication if something is wrong with your current plan and allow you to make any modifications before it's too late.

your training instead. As a coach, Glassford says that he often sees clients fretting over weight loss when they could easily see faster and more effective performance results by focusing on bike skills, preparation, mental skills, following a proper training plan, and eating well.

So before you continue, it's important to be clear on why you want to lose weight—don't assume that getting lighter is the only way to improve your cycling, especially if you're already close to your optimal racing weight.

## HOW DO I LOSE WEIGHT?

Fad diets come and go, but the secret to losing weight is actually incredibly simple, no matter which diet you're talking about. "Being in a calorie deficit is what's required," explains Guest. "All fad diets ultimately lead to caloric deficit, and that's why they work." But the calorie deficit is usually not sustainable and the weight comes back.

"The best thing we can manipulate is calories in," she explains. "Most people can't train enough to make a 500-calorie deficit—that's most practically achieved by eating less while exercising a bit more. Since cyclists on specific training plans can't always change up how much they burn, let's focus on what we can control instead."

But skipping meals isn't the answer, especially if you lead an active lifestyle. "If you keep cutting calories, your body adapts. This is metabolic adaptation: The metabolic and physiological changes that occur during weight loss decrease your energy needs as you lose weight, so you have to keep eating less and less to be in a calorie deficit. You've heard before how the body goes into starvation mode for survival. The science is a little more complex, but that's basically it," Guest says. "It turns into a hibernating bear that can go the winter on very few calories, and that's how metabolism slows down. It's the body's defense.

"People are always thinking about burning more fat as their main fuel source while exercising, but that absolutely doesn't translate into losing body fat," she explains. "It takes a caloric deficit so the body taps into body-fat stores." The idea is to burn more calories than you take in to create a caloric deficit, which your body will make up for by burning fat.

"If you go to bed with a 500-calorie deficit, even though you've only burned carbs all day in a sprint workout, then overnight your body will have to dip into body-fat stores to use as a fuel for the bodily functions that would have been fueled by the carbohydrates you already burned," she explains. "At the end of the day, as long as you've depleted those calories, your body will have a high percentage of energy coming from fat when you're sleeping.

"What's important is that calorie deficit if you're trying to burn body fat," she concludes. "As long as you burn calories, you'll drop body fat—your body has to break the body fat down to use for the energy needs of nonexercise energy-requiring bodily functions, from muscle repair to hormone production to brain function to growing hair and toenails."

Pro cyclocrosser Katie Compton puts Guest's words into practice when it's time to drop a pound or two to get to race weight for the season. "I just count calories," Compton says. "I don't keep a perfect tally, but between my SRM power data measuring device (calculates calories burned in-ride) and my resting metabolic rate, I have a good idea of how many calories I burn. And once you measure out your food a couple of times, you start learning what 3 ounces of meat looks like and how many calories are in it. You know what a cup of rice looks like and how many grams of carbohydrates are in it.

"Weight loss comes back to knowing what you're putting out—doing things like using an app like MyFitnessPal to track what you eat and what you do in a day," explains pro cyclocrosser Jeremy Powers. "If you're cutting 500 calories a day, you probably won't even notice."

Of course, calorie restriction comes with a few caveats. First, Guest warns, "the more you restrict, the higher your risk for bingeing." If you go to bed hungry every night, you're more likely to sneak in that chocolate bar at midnight or opt for a second helping of pancakes in the morning. Pay close attention to your mood since restricting constantly can make you miserable and no fun to be around, on the bike or off.

Second, don't shave off calories where you need them the most: during your ride. Focus your calorie restriction to times not directly around your ride. As mentioned earlier, your ride is not the time to worry about losing an ounce or two. The idea is to lose weight in order to improve your performance, so why sabotage your performance in the process? It just doesn't make sense.

Third, constant calorie restriction can result

in a plateau for many athletes. Compton explains, "If you keep cutting calories and keep being hungry all the time, your body is eventually going to just slow down and lower your metabolism and you'll stop losing weight. But if you cut 200 to 300 calories a day most days and take a day or two a week where you eat normally, you'll slowly lose weight and keep your metabolism up. Just fuel with healthy foods."

You may want to count calories 1 or 2 days a week, but you don't need to be a slave to your calories every day to see results. "The best approach if you're wanting to lose weight," Guest concludes, "is to exercise a bit more and eat a bit less, but not do anything dramatic. Look at how clothes fit, how your belt tightens. We tend to deposit the most fat around the middle, so that's a good gauge. We have the ability to quantify a lot of things—calories in certain foods, calories taken in—but I don't know that it's always useful."

To cut calories without impacting your training, try shifting your perspective of what a traditional day is. "When I work with athletes, they can't afford to have a sub-optimal training session," Guest says. "I have them meet their caloric needs every day, but then I'll take advantage of working around their rest days to lose body fat."

What does she mean? "Say you have a Saturday morning training session, but Sunday is a rest day. You want your training and recovery meals on Saturday morning and early afternoon, before and after your ride, but starting at 3:00 p.m., the rest of the day is your 'diet' day because you don't have to fuel your Sunday rest day," she says. That doesn't mean fasting, but it does mean calorie restriction without compromising your training.

"This way, you can get into a caloric deficit and with an additional 500 or more calories off on Saturday night. Then on Sunday, you want to use the first half of the Sunday to stay in that deficit and take off another 500 calories—now you're in deficit of 1,000 extra calories. But Sunday, later in the afternoon and night, you want to go back to normal because you need to fuel Monday's training," Guest explains.

**Creating a calorie deficit over a 24-hour period is much less painful** when it's afternoon to afternoon since you get full meals each day but you're still creating a day's worth of caloric cutbacks.

"So there's a half-day Saturday and Sunday where you can create a deficit and it won't impact recovery or training," she concludes. "That has really worked over a longer period, steadily inching toward losing 1 pound a week and trying to get most of that pound off in one deficit day. It's how you can trick the body into letting go of half a pound of fat in a 24-hour period while still having a solid training week, even with 24 hours of dramatic caloric restriction."

Sneaky, right? There have been countless studies on the various dietary approaches to healthy, sustainable weight loss, but the research is often confusing. The truth is, there are many different strategies, but one must be aware of how much weight (pardon the pun) should be placed on each parameter of effort when modifying your diet for weight loss or changes in body composition.

Seventy percent of weight loss is based on the simple balance of calories in and calories out. "Restriction of energy intake is the primary method of producing a negative energy balance leading to weight loss," explains Guest. "About 70 percent of your efforts belong here. If you don't eat less, you won't lose, period! Calories are your weapon to lose fat."

Twenty percent of weight loss is related to how your body metabolizes the three macronutrients. "Diets of similar overall energy content but with different macronutrient distribution can affect metabolism, appetite, and thermogenesis in different ways," explains Guest. The main thing to remember is to hit that optimal protein number and use carbohydrates as fuel for training. The other 10 percent is outside factors: things like how well you're sleeping, how you're training, and when you're eating.

Keep in mind that everyone is different, and it's up to you to experiment. "Some evidence suggests differences in individual responses to diets are associated with specific genotypes," says Guest. "So looking at your DNA is in the near future when it comes to assessing the influence of macronutrient composition on weight management and/or weight loss."

What about supplements? Caffeine may help you work harder, but anything else out there that promises to help you lose weight likely has dangerous side effects—and is potentially illegal. (For more information, see Chapter 16.)

## KEEP IT CLEAN

At the end of the day, healthy foods will eventually get you to where you want to go, as long as you're smart about it. Calorie counting is a lot less painful when you're still feeling full, thanks to the satisfying salad you had for lunch, filled with clean and nutritious calories.

Pro mountain biker Georgia Gould breaks it down by bluntly saying: "Listen to your body. And think less crap, more good food. Think about if you're full. Even if it's delicious, if you're full, stop eating."

Her secret to keeping herself full and in prime racing shape is simple: "Even when I'm not eating as clean as I could be, I'm still having a lot of fruits and vegetables. It's important that most of your diet is like that most of the time. Then you can veer off a little here and there. But for health and feeling good, a more whole-foods-heavy diet is key."

Nutritionist Jordan Dubé, MS, agrees wholeheartedly with Gould, saying, "if we eliminate processed carbs, take them completely off the table, and replace those with lots and lots of vegetables, fruits, and whole grains—not processed, but literal whole grains like brown rice, quinoa—that is usually enough to spark some change in a person."

Just adjusting some of our less-than-stellar food choices toward unprocessed, whole-foods options can create a positive shift for a lot of people. "That will create a caloric deficit because those foods aren't calorically dense, they haven't been chopped up and put back together as something processed, so you'll actually eat more volume but end up in a calorie deficit," Dubé explains. "They also last longer and take longer to digest, so you're not hungry as often. Processed food with sugar tends to produce cravings and reduce tastebuds' ability to appreciate naturally sweetened foods like fruit. So if you cut out the processed stuff, you won't be constantly craving processed carbs."

Another overlooked element is how much water we're drinking. Simply being aware of our hydration can make a huge difference when it comes to how hungry we feel and how alert we are during the day. "Hydration status is really important for weight loss," adds Dubé. "So many people are chronically dehydrated, especially athletes. So making sure you're consuming enough water throughout the day is really important."

To make sure you're drinking enough, Dubé explains: "The best marker is urine color—light yellow. But if you're feeling tired all the time, that's a sign of dehydration as well. And if you feel hungry at a time of day when you normally wouldn't, rather than reaching for a snack, reach for a glass of water." (For information on urine testing, see the Appendix: Testing on page 191.)

"A lot of times, your brain recognizes signals of thirst as hunger," she adds. "So then people are eating when they're actually thirsty—and you can get water from the foods you eat, but it's so much easier to just drink a glass of water. So that can cut back on consumption as well—if you feel hungry, drink a glass of water, and if you still feel hungry after that, then eat something. But try a drink first."

## SUPERDIET: THE ANTI-SUPERFOOD

For my entire life, I've read article after article touting the new superfood. The food of the moment was often hard to come by, expensive, and ultimately, not that much better than its cheaper, more-common brethren. Goji berries, for example, had their moment, but blueberries, raspberries, and strawberries all have similar nutrient profiles. Coconut water was hailed as innovative and life changing 5 years ago but is now practically relegated to the same level as soft drinks, as more and more people realize how much sugar it contains despite the fact that it is labeled all-natural.

That isn't to say all popular superfoods are bad. Kale is a great leafy green option, and almonds—in raw and milk form—are wonderful as well.

The problem is when people become obsessed with these one-hit-wonder foods, they forget about all of the other options that exist. For instance, kale is fantastic, but people get kale obsessed and completely ignore spinach, romaine lettuce, Swiss chard, and plenty of other equally good options, and in doing so, they miss out on other key nutrients.

"There are no superfoods," says Nanci Guest, MSc, RD, CSCS. "It's more about whole foods versus processed foods. Foods that have had the least processing will be superior to other foods in most cases, but there's no magic food."

She explains, "Every year or two, people find a crazy new trend, like cacao or maca, and jump on it." While we have great new food options available, try to not obsess over them. "Instead of looking at things in isolation, look at them overall," she adds. "It's like training—your whole training. Look

## WATCH YOUR PORTIONS

For athletes—especially hungry ones after a long ride—it can be hard to keep a good handle on portion sizes. Eating at restaurants or even just pouring yourself a big bowl of cereal can easily sneak in calories, even if you're meticulous about recording them. How often have you actually weighed or measured that cup of oats you're about to make? Have you ever looked at the serving size on that big container of yogurt and measured out each scoop carefully? Over time, these little extras—a few grams here and there—can add up, even if we think we are tracking those calories.

"I see this problem with diet records all the time," says Guest. "Someone will say they had a bowl of oatmeal and a glass of juice. I'm like, at your whole diet, over months and years instead of day to day, because that's what's impacting you in the long term." You wouldn't do the same workout every single day to make progress, right? So why would eating one food be any better?

"A lot of these micronutrients are integrated into your cells over time, so it's the rating of your nutrient intake over weeks and months that matters," Guest explains. "You should aim for the superdiet of a variety of healthy foods versus thinking that eating one specific thing every day will make you healthy."

If there is no superfood, then what is a superdiet? Simple. "It's just a lot of variety—local, organic, nonprocessed foods—that's what will make a superdiet," Guest says. "Variety is huge—you can't just eat broccoli every day and that's it. You have to emphasize a variety of fruits and vegetables. Every plant food has hundreds of nutrients, and maybe 10 percent of them are unique to that food. Look at an almond and a walnut: They're similar but still have hundreds of nutrients that are different from each other, so you want to have the walnut and the almond, not just one or the other. So many people think nuts are good for them, but they only ever eat almonds because they're the ones mentioned in the news the most."

So take the superfood lists with a grain of salt, and eat some spinach the day after you go kale crazy.

And sorry, but chocolate—dark or not—isn't a health food when you eat a massive bar every night.

'Was that a half-cup of oatmeal? A full cup? How many ounces of juice?' Everyone's bowl is different. That's why you need a consistent measurement to give you a real portion size."

Even worse is when you're not in charge of your own food preparation, especially when eating out. "You have these super-size sodas and giant muffins and all-you-can-eat buffets, and that's when carbs become the problem," says Guest. "People are overestimating what a serving is." Not only do people overestimate serving size and calories, but it's hard to even ascertain what the exact ingredients are. You don't know how much oil went into that sauce, and there's no way to measure exactly how much pasta you're eating. Just be aware that when you eat out, it's most likely a bigger serving than the one you're logging into your calorie counter.

Eating at restaurants or with friends is often one of the more challenging times to stick to a healthy meal plan. "When dieting, it's good practice to warn people," says Powers. "Tell them, 'I'm on a serious diet right now' if you're going out. But it's pretty commonplace to have a lot of restrictions right now—for example, people know I don't eat dairy when I'm coming over."

## PERIODIZATION OF WEIGHT LOSS

If you want to train and race like the pros, consider one of their strategies of getting to race weight through nutrition periodization, which is where your dietary and nutritional habits mirror your training to achieve peak performance at a specific time of the year. With nutrition periodization, you are at peak race weight for important races, but it's okay to let the reins slip a little in the off-season. It's not a green light to pack on 20 pounds, but an extra piece of pie in November when your next race isn't until June is completely fine, and it can even save your sanity.

"You may want to plan weight loss around peak performance," says Glassford, who pushes himself and his riders to find that balance. "We're starting to understand how racing weight is key, but we don't see people focusing on it in cycling. So you can cut in the short term, but if you start seeing a performance decline then it isn't worth it. If the power to weight isn't increasing with weight loss, that's a problem. I've seen lots of riders who pushed race weight for too long—I've done it myself. I was light, but my threshold didn't increase for a few years. Then I gained a few pounds and gained a lot of watts and much better overall health. It's hard in cycling, because there's the belief that being at your lightest is always the answer."

He adds, "Periodization of nutrition strategy has been huge. So if you're in a base training period, you're doing lower intensity and so your carbohydrate needs aren't as high. You can lower carbs, possibly go a bit higher in fat.

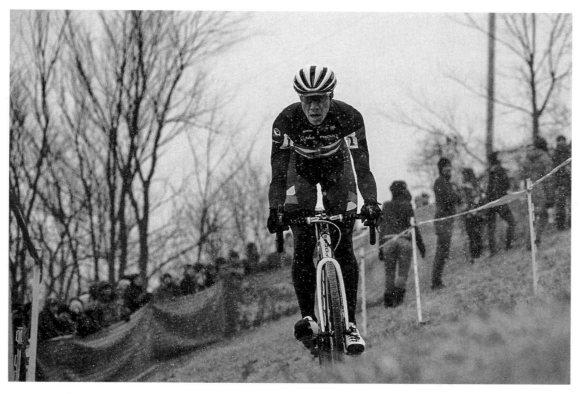

Pro cyclocrosser Jeremy Powers focuses on his race weight during the season but does loosen the reins a bit in the off-season.

You could run the tank a little lower in rides. But as race season and higher-intensity workouts come in, you need to add a few more carbs. So making people understand that nutrition isn't the same all year is huge."

If you want to drop weight, try to do so before race season, so you can focus on performance during key points of the season. In short, limit indulgences after races and make sure to take in enough good carbs and protein to properly recover so you're ready for the next effort.

After the race season is over, you can loosen your belt (figuratively and literally) for a couple of months to protect your sanity and enjoy your favorite foods. Just be sure to eventually refocus your diet and get back into peak race shape for the seasonal cycle to begin again.

"Riders always want to be at their skinniest, all year long, but it never works out like that," says Powers. "You get skinny, then throughout the season, you gain a little bit of weight while racing, then lose it again, then gain it back. It's like constant do-overs. You won't be at perfect race weight all year long if you're constantly on the road racing and traveling a ton."

Because of this constant flux, Powers says, "I'm a big fan of tracking to see what you're getting. A lot of people think they're getting something and aren't."

That said, Powers does take a break from counting calories to indulge a bit in the off-season before cleaning up to race again. "I don't log calories every day, but there are times of year when I know I'm putting out this amount of calories, and I know I want to lose weight so I need to know what my calorie intake is."

In addition to an annual nutrition periodization, you can also segment your nutrition and calorie counting on a weekly basis. Mini lows and highs throughout the week can actually help you drop weight faster, as those higher-calorie days keep your metabolism revved up. Too many days in caloric deficit can lower your base metabolic rate, which may cause you to retain or even gain weight. So, live a little, but be smart. "It depends what your goals are," Guest explains. "Have your strict day, but have those days that are a bit more relaxed. And that supports not having metabolic resistance.

"If we look at the guidelines of needing, say, 3,000 calories a day if you're training every day," she elaborates, "to lean out, do 2,500 per day but go back up to 3,000 one or two days a week. You wouldn't train intensely every day of the week, so why would you eat the same every day?"

As mentioned earlier, don't use your rest days as splurge days. Plan your indulgences around bigger or harder training sessions, and keep your calories low on your days off the bike when you don't need as much energy. "It's so important to feed your training," says Guest. "A rest day isn't the time to do a splurge day."

Let's clarify one thing: When we say splurge, we mean an extra 200 to 500 calories in a day. "Big cheat days derail you to a much higher extent," warns Guest. "If you consume an extra 2,000 calories on Sunday, Monday through Friday end up much harder because you went so overboard that you're that far behind."

Competitive cyclists should experiment with a nutrition periodization strategy based on their training and race calendar, while those looking to slim down should try a weekly approach. And no matter what, keep any indulgences small if weight loss is truly your goal.

## CARBS, PROTEIN, AND FAT

In a recent nutrition review, J. Alfredo Martinez co-director of the Institute of Food and Nutritional Sciences at the University of Navarra in Pamplona, Spain, writes that caloric restriction is the primary way to create negative energy (calorie deficit) in the quest for weight loss. But that doesn't mean macronutrient distribution doesn't play an important role. When looking to lose those last couple of pounds, you may need a little extra push to reach your goal race weight. However, you risk lowering your energy and power levels by cutting even more calories, so dialing in little things like nutrient breakdown and adjusting ratios can help.

First, consider raising your protein intake and reducing carbohydrates. This doesn't mean low carb, by any stretch. Carbohydrates will still be your primary fuel for riding, but up your protein to hit at least 20 grams in each meal, four times a day. "High protein is good because it helps maintain lean muscle and keeps you more satisfied," Guest explains.

Martinez cites a study of nearly 7,000 overweight women who were divided into groups based on four caloric-restriction diets: The first group exercised and followed a diet with a 1:1 ratio of carbohydrates to protein; the second group exercised and followed a diet with a 1:3 ratio of carbohydrates to protein; the third and fourth groups followed the same nutrient breakdown but without exercise. Three months later, the women in the high-protein-diet-plus-exercise group had lost an average of 15.5 pounds, while the 1:1 protein-to-carb group, also exercising, lost only 4.6 pounds, on average.

"There seems to be evidence that you can go really high protein, protect your muscle mass, and not be hungry because you can consume a lot of calories, but you can still lose weight," says Guest. "You don't gain as much weight consuming extra protein compared to fat or carbs."

While raising your protein intake is an effective way to lose weight, don't skip the carbs altogether, and be careful not to add fat to your diet as you increase protein. "The best experts in the world are still really pro carb," says Guest.

If you already claim to be low carb, you may not be as low as you think. "A lot of people think that they're going low carb, but really, most aren't," she adds. "I hear all the time, 'I don't eat sugar,' or 'I don't eat carbs but I eat fruit.' People are confused by what carbs are. Sugars, fruit, vegetables, grains—there are carbs in almost everything other than pure animal protein."

As an athlete, you can still cut back on carbohydrates because you may not be aware of how many carbs you actually consume. "A lot of recreational people tend to overfuel their rides—especially cyclists who aren't riding every day," says Glassford. If you're not riding every day, you don't need to carb-load, you don't need a high-carb diet."

"A lot of people don't recognize how many carbs are in different things," Guest adds,

## GETTING OVER THE PLATEAU

Think cutting calories is the only way to achieve your ideal body composition? You may be wrong—and if you've been hitting a plateau no matter how many calories you cut, you may actually need to eat more to see a positive change. Sounds crazy, but when restricting calories, our metabolisms actually slow down to match the caloric intake—so starving yourself may be the exact wrong thing to do.

In a recent study in the *International Journal of Exercise Science* that focused on a female collegiate cross-country team, a nutritionist gave the runners a new diet plan for a 4-week trial—the plan increased caloric intake by around 400 calories per day—and within 8 weeks, the women saw a slight decrease in body fat and positive change in their bone mineral density.

echoing Glassford's sentiments. "Like at Starbucks, they have banana loaf, and people are unaware that you can pack 500 calories and over 50 grams of carbs into that small piece of bread." You may not be aware of how many carbs you consume on a daily basis, whether you consider yourself low carb or not. By simply identifying and eliminating the extra carbs in your diet, you can reduce your daily caloric intake—being aware of what you're eating is half the battle when it comes to weight loss. Once you start to realize how many calories, especially in carbohydrate form, you're eating in a day, you may realize you're taking in a lot more than you really need.

Guest is a major proponent of carbohydrates in an athlete's diet, but even she admits that if the scale won't budge, cut carbs. "If an athlete is having a hard time losing that last couple percent of body fat or last couple pounds, going a little lower and cutting back carbs is what they need to do," she says. "But it doesn't need to be low carb exactly, it just means cutting back on carbs and adding a bit more protein."

Martinez writes between 25 and 75 percent of body weight variability is influenced by genetics. That's a lot we can't control. But genetic testing, which can give us a better idea of the best macronutrient breakdown for our specific genetic makeup, is becoming more common and readily available (see Chapter 18 for more information).

For the rest of us, it comes back to whole foods and a steady but small caloric deficit to drop weight over time.

## STILL NOT LOSING?

If the number on the scale just won't budge and your body-fat percentage still hasn't dropped, no matter how clean your diet is or how much you've been riding, you may need to eat more.

I'll pause for a second while you celebrate.

Guest gives an example, citing some of the athletes she's worked with in the past as she's prepped racers for the Olympics, the Pan American Games, and through her personal-training business. "You have three similar people expending 3,000 calories a day," she starts. "But one of them is eating what she's burning, while the other two are in deficit. And while that might have caused weight loss initially, over time, the deficit creates a metabolic shift, so the women eating less are getting negatively impacted, both in terms of their body-fat percentages and their overall health," Guest explains. "So, what we've seen is the person eating 3,000 calories a day will have the lowest body fat while the one in the greatest deficit will have higher body fat," Guest concludes, adding that the person at the greatest deficit

also runs the risk of other negative side effects, like frequent illness, anemia, and loss of menstrual periods.

Sound counterintuitive? The body is resilient and works hard to adjust to what it's dealing with. Therefore, a constant calorie restriction, especially one that large, will eventually hurt you and put your entire well-being at risk, even more so if you're training at a high volume. "The body can adapt and be shifting energy away from reproduction—so you're losing your period—and taking away from immunity or proper recovery. This is where we see overtraining and frequent illness," explains Guest.

"In the personal training and endurance world," Guest says, "we're constantly telling people to get leaner you have to eat more. That concept came from the bodybuilding world, and it was really eye-opening."

Unfortunately, there is no magic secret to immediate weight loss. "You have to be strategic and lose weight slowly," Guest concludes. "Doing it fast just doesn't work. To drop 5 pounds, you'll be more successful dropping a pound a week for 5 weeks. I tell

| | WEIGHT | CALORIES BURNED | CALORIES EATEN | BODY FAT (%) |
|---|---|---|---|---|
| Person 1 | 130 lb | 3,000 | 3,000 | 15 |
| Person 2 | 130 lb | 3,000 | 2,500 | 17 |
| Person 3 | 130 lb | 3,000 | 2,200 | 20 |

clients, 'You have to be sneaky about it, and you have to be strategic so you trick the body into not feeling any pressure or that there's any harm. We're designed to survive, and the survival mechanism is to hoard calories, feast or famine.'"

Losing weight slowly allows your body to drop fat rather than muscle. And no, you don't want to lose muscle. Therefore, testing body-fat percentage regularly versus hopping on the scale can provide a more accurate measurement of how your body is reshaping itself. But keep in mind that everyone is different, and there are benefits to regular weigh-ins, as mentioned earlier.

"Because cyclists don't have to use a lot of power, they can do without a lot of lean muscle," Guest says, but adds, "that leaves them open to becoming 'skinny fat,' where they have a higher level of body fat but little lean muscle mass."

Lean muscle mass doesn't mean you'll ride slower because you're weighed down. Some lean muscle is only going to aid your riding, and—on a completely shallow note—will look healthier and better than that string bean, skinny-fat physique. "Some people want to be great athletes," Guest says, "but they also want to look good."

Lastly, if you're having trouble losing weight and hitting the body-fat percentage you're aiming for, consider toning up by adding some strength and core training to your routine. Adding more lean muscle mass can make a diet work for you if hours on the bike and dieting just won't cut it. "You can lean out and get rid of extra body fat by adding a bit of extra-lean muscle," says Guest. "That seems to shift metabolism and help to lean out the abdomen. Strength training just seems to help lean out that visceral—abdominal—fat."

# YOUR FIVE TAKEAWAYS

1. Regular weigh-ins can help you stay on track, but also pay attention to your body-fat percentage and your power numbers to gauge progress.

2. Low-level caloric restriction is the simplest, most-efficient way to drop weight.

3. Periodize your nutrition: Enjoy the off-season and indulge a bit. Just be sure to refocus and hit your ideal weight right before race season and maintain it throughout the season.

4. Don't restrict calories every day: Have days where you hit your needs (or even indulge by 200 to 500 extra calories) to keep your metabolism stoked.

5. To drop those difficult last few pounds or body-fat percentage points, slightly raise your protein intake and lower your carbohydrates—but don't go low or no carb!

# CHAPTER FIFTEEN

# STRESS, FOOD INTOLERANCE, AND THE CYCLIST

When it comes to feeling your best, training your hardest, and avoiding unwanted weight gain, you can't rely on diet alone. We all know we are what we eat but how we eat also plays a huge role in how we feel. Environmental factors beyond what we actually consume can affect our overall health and well-being.

The secret sabotage from stress and lack of sleep can be an athlete's worst nightmare. Unfortunately, high stress and lack of sleep seem to be the norm for the busy athlete. Whether you're just juggling a lot (working full-time, raising a family, maintaining a training plan) or you're terrified during race week (worrying about the what-ifs of race day), stress and sleep have a huge impact on your life and, when not managed correctly, can often wreak havoc on your system, diet or no diet.

Let's start with sleep. In 2014, Jan Machal, a researcher at Masaryk University in the Czech Republic, published a paper on sleep disturbances and their relationship with food-intake disorders and found that reduced sleep time causes unhealthy food choices and weight gain. Unfortunately, people who don't live by a circadian rhythm (sleep when it's dark, wake up when it's light) are at risk for unhealthy metabolic shifts and possible psychological issues such as "night eating syndrome," where eating at night is a mental necessity, Machal argues.

Of course, as we balance work, life, family, training, and a multitude of other things, our daytime activities often run into the evening hours, and this can affect both the quantity and quality of our sleep. How many times have you gotten up when it's still dark out to hop on the trainer or gone for a group ride as the sun was setting in the summer?

In addition to packing on pounds, a lack of sleep can also be an athletic inhibitor. According to a recent study from the *Journal of Pediatric Orthopaedics*, young athletes who chronically missed out on sleep were more susceptible to injury on the playing field.

Some people need only 6 hours of sleep per night, and some athletes won't function well with under 10. Unfortunately, there's no golden number. To find out how much you need, consider keeping a journal to note how many hours you slept and jot down a quick summary of how you felt and how your training went. After a few weeks, you should be able to see patterns emerge and you can zero in on your ideal number—typically somewhere between 7 and 9 hours.

In addition to lack of sleep, stress can also have a negative impact on your health. Nanci Guest, MSc, RD, CSCS, has seen a higher injury-to-stress ratio. "I did my master's work on cognitive dietary restraint and stress fractures in female runners," she explains. "According to a survey that these women completed, the runners all ate similarly, but the ones with high dietary restraint (the ones that actually limited what they ate, logged what they ate, and ate only a certain number of calories), despite taking in the same amount of calories as the people without diet restraint, had higher levels of stress hormones like cortisol, and that's what was affecting their menstrual cycles and bone health and, therefore, raised their potential for stress fractures."

So, despite the fact that the women were all eating similar diets, those who spent time fretting about every calorie actually raised their overall stress levels, which created significant health risks. "Worrying about what you're eating is affecting you as much as what you are eating," says Guest. "In my stress factor group, the higher-stress group was only different because of their dietary restraints."

"I don't necessarily find that stress impacts my digestion," says retired pro cyclocrosser Mo Bruno Roy. That may be because as a yoga instructor and cyclocross racer, she's incredibly calm and channels her emotions into racing. "I try to keep my stress levels low," she says but adds that stress can often come in the form of travel—a common problem for those of us balancing the business world and a cycling habit.

"Travel impacts my digestion, because I find that I just don't get hungry as often," she explains. Her problem isn't eating junk food at airports, though. It's a problem less frequently mentioned when it comes to travel-associated stress: weight loss. "That's hard in cyclocross season—I just don't eat! And if you lose 2 to 3 pounds in the season, that's 10 watts. I find it happens more when it's cold out. You do an intense workout or race, and it's cold and you just aren't hungry. You end up drinking a smoothie that just has 400 calories, and maybe some dinner later, but you don't really want it. I just end up opposed to food, in general—nothing is appealing. So I need to make sure I have foods that I really want around me so I do want to eat."

## STRESS AND FOOD INTOLERANCES

Picture this scene for a minute: You've had a really hard, stressful week. You've put in big training hours because you have a race next weekend, your boss is on your back about a really critical project, your kid is having a hard time in school, and your significant other is upset because of your time spent on the bike. Your stomach is likely tied up in knots by the time you get home on Thursday night. It's too late to make dinner, so you decide to order a pizza (with extra vegetables, at least!). You chow down on five slices (you had a hard ride earlier) while you watch TV, then get in a shouting/barking match with the dog. An hour later, your stomach is killing you.

Does your stomach hurt because you're gluten-intolerant? Are you lactose-intolerant? Are you allergic to those mushrooms? Or are you just stressed out and your stomach hurts because you housed five slices in record time and your gut is just trying to catch up?

More and more people are self-diagnosing food intolerances of all kinds, and while most

have some basis for self-diagnosing, there's a certain level of hypochondria out there as well. Crazy enough, though, believing that you have a food intolerance can quickly become a self-fulfilling prophecy.

"There are some interesting studies coming out surrounding perceived food intolerances, like lactose intolerance," says Guest. "There's a study where people who are self-reported as lactose-intolerant were given what they were told was lactose, but it was actually a lactose-free placebo. So they thought they were getting lactose and were able to produce the symptoms of intolerance without actually having it. You can create bloating, cramping, and diarrhea with your mind. That totally complicates things."

If you believe you have a food intolerance, avoid self-diagnosing and discuss it with your doctor. That said, avoiding lactose or gluten, as long as the substitutes are healthy whole foods instead of engineered fake versions, is completely fine from a health perspective.

Throughout this book, we've heard from pro road racer Tayler Wiles, who largely eats gluten-free in deference to her partner with celiac disease; Bruno Roy, who follows a vegan diet; and pro cyclocrosser Jeremy Powers, who refuses to eat anything processed.

Pro cyclocrosser Katie Compton is one athlete who makes a healthy diet possible within the confines of her otherwise debilitating allergy to histamines and gluten intolerance.

## DO YOU HAVE A FOOD INTOLERANCE?

Because gluten-free eating is the hot-button trend at the moment, it's easy to jump on the gluten-sensitivity bandwagon. But if you're experiencing a lot of digestive upset, it may not be the cause.

There aren't any medical tests that pinpoint intolerances (such as for allergies or celiac disease); therefore, the fastest way to self-diagnose is through an elimination diet. One of the best ways is with the Fermentable Oligosaccharides, Disaccharides, Monosaccharides, and Polyols (FODMAPs) diet, as Nanci Guest, MSc, RD, CSCS, explains.

"Not sure if gluten is your issue? Well, for 95 percent of us, it's not," she says. "Recent research showed that many suffering from non-celiac gluten sensitivity (or NCGS, for short) are actually more sensitive to FODMAPs, and not gluten, per se. Data from a recent study suggest that NCGS might not be a discrete entity, and gluten might be not be a specific trigger of gastrointestinal symptoms once dietary FODMAPs are reduced."

So what exactly are FODMAPs, other than a slightly hilarious acronym? "FODMAPs are carbohydrates that may be poorly absorbed in the small intestine of some people. FODMAPs move through the digestive tract to the large intestine, where they can draw water into the colon and are rapidly digested by naturally occurring gut bacteria," explains Guest. "The fermentation of FODMAPs produces gas and other by-products. While some people are able to consume FODMAPs without experiencing gastrointestinal side effects, many people with digestive disorders, such as irritable bowel syndrome (IBS), find that FODMAPs trigger symptoms including abdominal pain, cramping, bloating, excess gas, constipation, and/or diarrhea."

She has battled plenty of digestive issues over the years before arriving at the diet she currently enjoys—and a diet that propelled her to more than 10 National titles.

"Within the last 10 years, I've tried a bunch of different things—from counting carbohydrates to counting protein to the macronutri-

ents and how many grams I need to how to lose weight to nutrient timing, and dealing with my allergies and food intolerances," she recalls. "I've tweaked my diet a lot over the last decade, especially the last couple of years. I have really bad allergies—seasonal allergies and food intolerances that affect my allergies. So, I actu-

Unfortunately, the FODMAPs diet eliminates of a lot of food, including the following:

- Fructose (fruit, honey, high-fructose corn syrup)
- Lactose (dairy)
- Fructans (wheat, garlic, onion)
- Galactans (legumes, including beans, lentils, soybeans)
- Polyols (sweeteners containing isomalt, mannitol, sorbitol; plus stone fruits like avocados, cherries, nectarines, peaches)

So, if you have a lot of stomach upset (diarrhea, constipation, gas, bloating and/or cramping) or have been diagnosed with IBS or gluten intolerance, you may want to consider looking into a FODMAPs elimination diet. Keep in mind that this diet is not for everyone, and those without food intolerances will not benefit from eliminating these foods.

Even those following a FODMAPs diet can opt for a moderate approach and just cut back on the foods listed. But for those wanting to follow the process exactly, there are plenty of websites with the full list of foods on the do and don't eat list. The process involves eliminating all of the foods containing FODMAPs for 6 weeks, and then gradually adding them back in—one at a time—noting if any cause gastrointestinal distress. You may find that gluten is the culprit, but you may be surprised and find that it's actually lactose that's giving you problems, or that high-fructose corn syrup needs to be out of your diet entirely.

It's not easy, but if you do have persistent stomach problems, this diet will help target the culprits.

ally recently started on a low-histamine diet, which isn't a typical diet you see. But I read a bunch of research on allergies and how to perform and eat without feeling awful, and now I eat foods that don't add histamines to my diet. Most people have no idea what high-histamine foods are, but they include a lot of smoked foods, cultured foods, fermented foods, wine, yeast, and certain vegetables. . . . I also have a grass allergy, so I stay away from wheat. It annoyingly eliminates enough foods to make it difficult."

She doesn't completely eschew histamines and occasionally indulges in some of her favorites, like chocolate and wine. But she does so in moderation. "And it helps; it makes a big difference for me," she adds.

Part of alleviating her diet stress, she says, was just coming to terms with her allergies and intolerances and accepting that certain foods make her feel bad. She can either avoid those foods altogether or recognize how they make her feel and move on. "If I eat wheat or cultured food, I'll feel shitty for a minimum of a week, because it takes my body that long to recover from the inflammation," she explains. "Whenever I eat something like that, I can tell, and I know I'll feel bad."

There is a psychological component, as the lactose-intolerance study showed: If we eat something knowing that it should make us feel terrible, the odds are good that we will, in fact, feel terrible. And why would you knowingly eat something that won't make you feel (and perform) at your best?

Bruno Roy recalls her struggles with learning what to avoid to keep stomach issues at bay: "When my sister and I went to college, and I was having difficulty digesting things, I think it was partially because I'd just spent 4 years in high school running competitive track constantly injured. It took a few years of chronic stomach pain and experimenting with different diets to straighten it back out. Now, I'm pretty picky; I don't do things that are spicy or super-oily or anything. And I definitely don't do new things during competition."

In short, before you remove a huge food group like gluten or lactose from your diet, you may want to consider if your intolerances are related to something else, like stress.

One way to gauge food sensitivities is to keep a food diary. If you log what you eat (and note if there's a certain time of day your stomach hurts), you can look back at your log and recognize patterns. Maybe your stomach bloats 3 hours after you eat something with dairy, or you tend to overindulge on chocolate right after conference calls with your boss. Knowing what your food sensitivities are and recognizing what triggers you to stress eat allows you to tailor your diet to cater to your individual needs. It's very hard to reach your performance goals when you constantly don't feel well.

That said, sometimes a food diary can add more stress to your day and to your eating, which is counterproductive. If that's the case, don't keep one for more than a day or two at a time. Just check in with how your macronutrients and calories are stacking up, and move on.

"Two or three times a year, I'll spend a day or two counting up my calories just to make sure I'm getting enough," explains pro road racer Janel Holcomb. "I add it up to see if I'm getting as much as I think I'm getting. Like, I'll make sure my breakfast is enough, I add it up and realize, 'Oh, okay, that's 1,000 calories in breakfast!'"

"I've done a food diary before, but I don't do

it anymore," says pro mountain biker Georgia Gould. "I gave the whole I'm-going-to-be-really-weird-about-my-diet thing a try, and it was miserable. I don't like having to write down everything and count all the calories and get totally wigged out about it."

Gould explains that focusing so intensely on what she's eating negatively impacts her, and since she's already a whole-foods-loving chef and a seasoned pro, she knows what her body needs. "Some people do really well being type A about that stuff and controlling it, but it makes me sad," she says. "I like cooking, I like food, and I don't like worrying about every little thing I eat."

Bruno Roy echoes her sentiment, saying, "You know what you need on a daily basis after a while. I know myself well enough that I don't need to write anything down, though I will occasionally go through a checklist in my head to make sure I ate enough of a certain thing that day."

Moral of the story? Keep calm and carry on. If your stomach hurts, pause for a minute and really think about what's making it hurt. You may find that stress is the culprit.

## YOUR FIVE TAKEAWAYS

1. Lack of sleep can be hard on your digestion—try to get 7 to 9 hours.

2. Stress about work, training, or especially about what you're eating, can have a negative impact on your digestion.

3. Thinking you have a food intolerance may cause stress, which can mimic the symptoms of actually having that intolerance.

4. If you think you have a food intolerance, keep a food diary to recognize any patterns, and talk to your doctor before self-diagnosing.

5. You can try cutting out things like gluten or dairy if it makes you feel better. Just be careful not to replace them with highly processed, less healthy versions.

# CHAPTER SIXTEEN

# SUPPLEMENTS

For athletes, maximizing performance and nutrition is always the goal. The assumption that taking a few supplements is a shortcut toward achieving optimal nutrient intake is why the supplement industry does so darn well. All of the supplements in the world, however, won't mitigate a poor diet. To state the obvious, they're called supplements for a reason: Ideally, they supplement and enhance an already stellar nutrient-dense diet.

"Quit looking for the shortcut or the magic bullet," says Nanci Guest, MSc, RD, CSCS. "Get away from supplements and processed foods. A lot of athletes don't even consider supplements. There's no downside to whole foods."

For those of you new to supplementing food with additional products, a supplement can be a vitamin or mineral, an herbal remedy or homeopathic medicine, muscle boosters or gainers, probiotics, fat burners, protein powders, and amino acids. But unlike food and pharmaceutical production, the supplement industry is subject to very little government regulation.

Consequently, supplements may include prohibited substances (intentionally or unintentionally because of cross-contamination during manufacturing), have inaccurately labeled ingredient lists, or make plenty of untrue claims. So choosing the right supplements can be tricky. We see from the high number of anti-doping violations that an athlete runs an extreme risk when using supplements. A positive doping test for an athlete who uses supplements may result in a violation regardless of how the prohibited substance got into the athlete's body, accidentally or on purpose.

However, there are some safe supplements that—when taken in conjunction with a good diet—can help keep the motor running as smoothly as possible. Just remember, "there's a mind-set that more is better, and you just don't have time to eat well," says Guest. "And I always say a poor diet with supplements is still a poor diet. You can't get away with having a crappy diet. There's no pill in the world

## COMPETITIVE CYCLISTS BEWARE

If you're a competitive cyclist, make sure that any supplement you take is 100 percent free of any banned substances. Check the World Anti-Doping Agency (wada-ama.org) or the NSF International Certified for Sport program's (nsfsport.com) websites for more information. Just remember that some sports supplements—despite what they say on the label—can test positive for banned substances. Be extremely careful of what you take, and as a rule, avoid anything with sports-enhancing claims.

Even if you're not worried about testing, tainted supplements can still be a problem. For example, supplements that promise muscle building may be tainted with steroids. In addition, many "fat burners" contain prescription weight-loss drugs and/or amphetamine derivatives, which can cause serious harm to your heart.

that's going to rescue you from having poor nutrition."

Be careful with what you put in your body. "Given enough time with any supplement,"

Guest adds, "we almost always see a problem, whether it's health or performance. We really have to rely on the body's ability to figure things out on its own."

Guest believes, however, that some supplements are useful, and sometimes even necessary, especially for athletes. "There are a few supplements that are warranted," she admits. For example, many female athletes need more iron due to the iron loss through their menstrual cycles and the trend toward consuming less red meat, which is a major source for heme, or high bioavailable iron. Likewise, the non-dairy trend has caused a need for supplemental calcium—the main mineral found in milk, cheese, yogurt, and other dairy products—in many of the athletes that Guest works with. Vegans and vegetarians need to be educated about balancing micronutrient intakes, while excluding most or all animal products and ensuring adequate calcium, iron, zinc, and vitamin $B_{12}$. "We may need more B vitamins for energy production; however, if you're eating more, you're automatically getting more B vitamins," she adds.

Nutritionist Jordan Dubé, MS, agrees and says, "Most supplements come with more risk than they're worth, unless you've been tested for deficiencies. Toxicity—having too much of something like iron—can be just as bad as a deficiency." She goes on to suggest that if you don't know for sure if you have a deficiency, you probably don't need that vitamin. A whole-foods diet should do the trick and, she explains, "If you're eating enough vegetables and whole grains, odds are you're getting those vitamins already. It might not be as high or concentrated as the quantities in a vitamin, but when they take foods apart and then glue them back together to make a supplement, it's not the same as coming from whole foods anyway. Plus, personal absorption rates vary a lot."

If your doctor does discover an imbalance in your blood panel and recommends taking a supplement, Dubé still believes that the ultimate solution doesn't just come in pill form. "I consider supplements temporary solutions until we can fix an athlete's diet," she says.

Guest echoes Dubé's sentiment, saying emphatically, "Supplements are just that—supplemental to a balanced diet." Some of us want the extra security that comes with popping a pill, though, and there are some supplements, like probiotics, that can be helpful regardless of what your daily diet looks like.

In the following pages, we take a look at the best supplements you can take without any harm. We break them down into two groups: lifestyle-enhancing vitamins and minerals, which claim to improve overall health, and ergogenic aids, which are designed to help you in training and adaptation. There are a few supplements that have been shown to improve

## SUPPLEMENTS FOR VEGETARIAN AND VEGAN ATHLETES

Iron deficiency is one of the most common nutritional deficiencies for vegetarian and vegan athletes, but make sure you actually need a supplement before you start taking one. Too much iron can create a toxic environment in your body, so have a blood panel done by your doctor prior to starting any kind of regimen.

"I take an iron supplement. It's not something you can often get enough of as an athlete," says vegan athlete and retired pro cyclocrosser Mo Bruno Roy, who regularly gets blood panels done to make sure she's in the proper iron range. She also adds that vegans should look closely at the macronutrients in their diets before adding supplemental soy, pea, or hemp protein to their regular nutrient intake.

Nutritionist Jordan Dubé, MS, adds, "I do recommend that clients are tested for deficiencies, and there are common ones like iron and B vitamins, especially among vegetarian and vegan athletes."

performance—but remember, none can come close to the benefits of being properly fueled from whole foods.

## VITAMINS AND MINERALS

**Multivitamins:** While your daily necessary vitamins should come from a diet rich in fruits and vegetables, taking a multivitamin every other day just to make sure you hit your target needs is perfectly fine. "My general approach is taking a multivitamin three times a week as a safeguard," says Guest. "But there's no reason to eat 100 percent of your needs from your diet and take 100 percent in a pill. That's just overkill, and it can lead to imbalances in things. We need such tiny amounts!"

**Vitamin D:** Getting a blood panel before beginning supplements of specific vitamins and minerals is advisable. Vitamin D, in particular, is one of the vitamins, as a cyclist, you should pay close attention to. Recent findings demonstrate how vitamin D is involved in the regulation of numerous skeletal and extraskeletal cellular processes that may underpin sports performance, making it an important part of our diets. Additionally, emerging evidence is finding that a vitamin D deficiency can have a profound effect on immunity, inflammation, and muscle function. Studies in athletic populations suggest that maintaining adequate vitamin D status may reduce stress fractures, total body inflammation, common

infectious illnesses, and impaired muscle function, and may also aid in recovery from injury.

Studies in athletes have found that vitamin D status varies among different populations and is dependent on skin color, early- or late-day training, indoor or outdoor training, and geographic location. The IOM recently classified the recommended daily dose of vitamin D status as roughly 600 IU a day, so make sure your supplement has that amount. Recommendations for exact amounts you should be supplementing are dependent on your current 25-hydroxyvitamin D prehormone concentration, which you can learn from your doctor. Vitamin D can also be obtained from regular safe sun exposure and dietary intake. Just be careful to avoid high dosages—if you're in the sun a lot, skip the vitamin D supplementation.

**Calcium:** "Make sure you have enough calcium. Having enough calcium and vitamin D in the diet is important," explains Guest. "This is important for cyclists. Calcium is important if you're not consuming dairy or are on a lower-calorie diet, where it can be hard to get in the quantity you need since you need a gram per day."

The IOM recommends 1,000 milligrams per day for adults and 1,200 milligrams per day for anyone over the age of 50.

Calcium is obviously important for bone health, but you can't rely on a supplement and diet to do all of the work. "You need an abnormal force to strengthen the bones," says Guest. "Running, for example, is not abnormal because your foot strikes the ground in a very repetitive, almost identical fashion . . . but things like hopping or squat jumps, where you land differently each time, will help, as will adding a bit of strength training." When you lift weights, the muscle pulls on either end of the bone while it contracts, which causes a slight bend in the bone and actually stimulates mineral (calcium) deposition into the bone to make it stronger to withstand the next bout of stress.

You may be concerned about high levels of protein and its ability to leach calcium away, but don't panic. "People worry that with high protein, the breakdown is too acidic, and you'll start bringing calcium out of the bones," says Guest. "But as long as you have enough fruits and vegetables, you'll have enough of an alkaline balance in the diet. Our body regulates acidity pretty well."

## ERGOGENIC AIDS

**Caffeine:** It's commonly known that coffee isn't just for the morning or an afternoon pick-me-up; it's helpful toward your performance in training and racing as well. In addition to traditional foods and beverages, caffeine is a common additive in sports-specific energy drinks and gels. According to Guest, some of the benefits include increased alertness and mood, as well as increased energy and concentration. In a recent study conducted by Robert Motl, PhD, at the University of Illinois at Urbana-Champaign, caffeine has also been shown to improve power, energy, and focus; to increase your pain threshold (great for those final, tough pushes); and to decrease your perceived effort levels.

There are downsides as well: The same crash that you experience when you skip breakfast and only have a cup of coffee (didn't

| DRINK | CAFFEINE (MG) |
|---|---|
| Starbucks coffee (20 oz) | 415 |
| Caffeine tablet (200 mg) | 200 |
| Dunkin' Donuts coffee (14 oz) | 178 |
| Starbucks espresso (2 oz) | 150 |
| McDonald's coffee (16 oz) | 133 |
| Maxwell House ground coffee (12 oz) | 100–160 |
| Black tea, brewed for 3 minutes (8 oz) | 30–80 |
| Mountain Dew (12 oz) | 54 |
| Coca-Cola (12 oz) | 35 |
| Red Bull (8.4 oz) | 80 |

you read the breakfast chapter?) is the same feeling you may experience in a workout or race fueled by caffeine: anxiety, increased heart rate, agitation, and nervousness (not great on the starting line). If you use caffeine to prep for a late-afternoon workout, it can also cause insomnia or restless sleep.

Caffeine isn't for everyone, so be sure to experiment with it before downing an energy drink right before a race or eating a caffeinated gel midride. People respond to caffeine differently, and certain genotypes (individuals with certain genetic makeups) experience a more positive impact.

A final benefit Guest adds is that "caffeine seems to be able to rescue the intensity of a fasted workout." Fasted state training is often tougher than a regular training session because—obviously—your glycogen stores are drained and you are feeling sluggish, so a bit of caffeine can make it more tolerable.

When supplementing caffeine, it doesn't take much to see the benefits. The accepted standard dose is 1.8 to 2.7 milligrams per pound of body weight. That's great news for those who want the performance benefits

| SUPPLEMENT | DOSAGE | TIMING | RESULTS |
|---|---|---|---|
| **Multivitamin** | 100% RDA | 3 times per week, depending on diet | Rounds out nutrition and avoids any chronic lack of a specific vitamin or mineral |
| **Probiotics** | 5 Billion+ CFU | Daily | Aid digestion and immunity by creating a happy and healthy microbiome filled with good gut bacteria |
| **Calcium** | 1,000 mg | Daily, depending on diet | Strengthens and improves bone health |
| **Vitamin D** | 600 IU | Daily in winter (get bloodwork for baseline) | Overall health, immunity, and muscle repair |
| **Creatine** | 3–5 g | Daily | Increases training volume and strength gains |
| **Caffeine** | 1.8–2.7 per lb of body weight | Pre-training or pre-race | Improves power, energy and focus; increases your pain threshold; and decreases your perceived effort levels |

*Note: All of these supplements are optional, but if you're interested in trying them, make sure to stay in the recommended dosage range.*

without the unfortunate side effects of being jittery or overstimulated that are often experienced in higher doses.

How much caffeine? We rounded up some of the more popular forms of caffeine so you can determine how many milligrams you're consuming on a daily basis. Use this information to plan your pre-ride amount perfectly.

**Creatine:** Creatine supplements have been shown to be effective at increasing high-intensity exercise capacity and improving muscle adaptation, but given its storied past, use caution when selecting your supplement to make sure it doesn't contain any banned substances.

Extensive research shows that oral creatine supplementation at a rate of 5 to 20 grams per day appears to be very safe and largely devoid of adverse side effects. Creatine works by rapidly resynthesizing adenosine triphosphate (ATP) from adenosine diphosphate (ADP) with the use of phosphocreatine (PCr) stored in muscles from supplementation. "This helps recover ATP more quickly after repeated sprints, while at the same time effectively improving the physiological response to resistance exercise, increasing the maximal force production of muscles in both men and women," Guest explains. "Basically, you can squeeze out two or three more reps at a given weight, which increases your volume of training without the extra effort and, therefore, improves strength gains." That might not

## WADA WEIGHS IN

The World Anti-Doping Agency (WADA) has an easy reference list of things that athletes should avoid to eliminate the risk of a positive drug test, as well as a list of supplements that they recommend as safe—and potentially beneficial.

Their no-fly list includes substances that are actually banned or have shown a high risk of contamination with substances that could lead to a positive drug test. The list includes ephedrine, strychnine stimulant, sibutramine, methylhexanamine (DMAA), dehydroepiandrosterone (DHEA), androstenedione, 19-Norandrosterone, Tribulus terrestris and other testosterone boosters, GH releasers and peptides, maca root powder, glycerol used for re-hyperhydration strategies, and colostrum (not recommended by WADA due to the inclusion of growth factors in its composition).

However, they do recommend iron supplements, as needed, as well as the previously discussed multivitamin, calcium and vitamin D, and probiotics to improve overall health. WADA also approves of caffeine and creatine as ergogenic aids, along with B-alanine, bicarbonate, and beetroot juice for potential fitness gains.

sound important for a cyclist, but think about how it could potentially impact your sprinting.

Thomas Buford of the International Society of Sports Nutrition (ISSN) claims that creatine is the most effective supplement for exercise and is potentially even useful for injury prevention. While it's impossible to say that it poses no long-term ill effects with 100 percent certainty—it's one of the most studied supplements, and it's been analyzed for long enough to be considered safe. Creatine is most effective when combined with protein and carbohydrate sources, so a post-ride smoothie would be the ideal time to add it to your nutritional repertoire.

For those of you who have never tried supplementing with creatine, the ISSN recommends starting with 3 days of about 15 to 20 grams, depending on body weight, and then cutting down to 3 to 5 grams (3 for lighter athletes, 5 for larger ones) per day to maintain elevated muscle creatine stores.

**Probiotics:** While not technically an ergogenic aid, probiotics can help athletes stay healthy and may have an impact on performance and recovery. In the last few years, pro-biotics have come into the public eye in a big way, and for good reason. Probiotics introduce good bacteria into your gut, and no matter how clean your diet is, adding them in can only help your digestion. "Probiotics are the one thing I really recommend," says Guest. "Taking them before breakfast is the best time, when your stomach is relatively empty.

"No one can dispute that you need healthy bacteria in your gut, so a probiotic can be helpful," she continues. "There's nothing definitive on what the best profile of bacteria is, so there's no perfect probiotic. But there are enough that we know are healthy, so I think most people can benefit from a probiotic. You'd have to eat five tubs of yogurt a day to get as much as you get from one probiotic in pill form since the pill versions contain billions of probiotics. And especially if you have a lot of immune system and gut problems, it becomes more important and helpful. Even colds and flus to cognition and mood are improved with probiotics." When shopping for a probiotic, look for one with at least 5 billion active cells.

# YOUR FIVE TAKEAWAYS

1. Supplements can't replace clean eating and should be taken in conjunction with a healthy diet. Be careful when choosing a supplement—look for quality sources that you trust. Use extra caution if you are a competitive cyclist to avoid risking a positive drug test.

2. Have your doctor take a blood panel to determine if you're low on any specific vitamins or minerals before dosing yourself with high levels of any supplement, especially iron.

3. A multivitamin three times a week can ensure that you are getting all essential nutrients, especially when supported by a healthy, wholesome diet with plenty of fruits and vegetables.

4. Caffeine can be a great ergogenic aid—but don't overindulge or you'll risk having uncomfortable side effects.

5. Creatine is accepted by most sports nutrition experts as a safe ergogenic aid that can improve muscle adaptation.

# CHAPTER SEVENTEEN

# IMMUNITY AND THE CYCLIST

You can't train if you're not healthy. Between a smart diet that fuels your body and provides plenty of vitamins and minerals—that same diet we've been talking about throughout the book—and a smart training plan that avoids falling into overtraining and fatigue, you should be pretty well covered. However, you can't be prepared for every eventuality, and unfortunately, athletes are not without certain levels of risk. Overtraining increases your risk of injury, and it can cause fatigue and make you sick. But there's also the risk of getting sick simply due to things like travel. We can't be 100 percent healthy all of the time, and even the toughest pro athlete gets sick. It's how you handle it that counts.

The most important thing to remember is that health should be your top priority and performance is secondary, according to Nanci Guest, MSc, RD, CSCS. You might be able to get in your training hours while sick or injured, but they likely won't be quality training hours that benefit your ultimate performance. If you're sick or injured, take a step back and assess how you're training—and fueling. "We're human beings before we're athletes," she says. "We want to think of health before performance, because the two are inextricably linked. You can't have consistently good performance without health. Training and competition over the long term requires a healthy body."

Sickness and injury can lead to interrupted training schedules, underperformance, or even missed competitions, so taking steps to increase your immunity before you're sick, and knowing how to handle your recovery if and when you do get sick or injured, is key.

That's why improving and maintaining a strong immune system is so important. Immunity, simply put, means having proper defenses to fight infection, disease, or viruses, in addition to minimizing inflammation and environmental sensitivities. Unfortunately, it's fairly easy to end up with a depressed immune function—particularly if you happen to be a high-performing athlete. Psychological stress, lack of sleep, and, of course, malnutrition can depress immunity, Guest explains.

You can easily fix any malnutrition issues by following the advice put forth in this book: balanced meals at the proper times, lots of fresh minimally processed foods, and proper in-ride fueling and hydration. But creating optimal sleep habits and minimizing stress are up to you.

## ILLNESS

During exercise, Guest explains, your exposure to airborne bacteria and viruses will increase as your breathing rate and depth is elevated—the standard response to riding hard on the bike. A rise in gut permeability (which is usually seen in endurance athletes because blood shifts away from the gut so frequently) may also introduce gut bacterial endotoxins into circulation, particularly during prolonged exercise in the heat. Additionally, as cyclists, we occasionally end up with cuts, scrapes, and road rash—another portal for bacteria. The exposure for novel bacteria is elevated when traveling, especially on planes or at races, where we're sur-

rounded by tons of people with new germs.

However, there are a few things you can do from a nutrition perspective to increase your immunity. First, make sure you're taking in adequate carbohydrates and staying hydrated, especially during exercise. Carbs decrease your inflammatory responses and limit the rise of stress hormones. "Carbohydrates suppress the release of cortisol, and since cortisol suppresses the immune function, it's important to include carbohydrates in your diet," explains Guest. Second, it's a good idea to take in carbohydrates in the form of a sports drink since dehydration can increase stress response and suppress the immune system.

Finally, make sure that your protein intake is adequate and frequent. If you're trying to lose weight and finding yourself constantly battling illness, consider increasing your daily intake since too little food can actually decrease your immune defenses. And if you have an immobilizing injury, get proper—and even slightly higher—doses of protein to prevent the loss of lean muscle mass from inactivity.

Another thing you can do to ward off illness is to add a probiotic to your daily routine, which we discussed in Chapter 16. This will improve microflora and enhance gut and systemic immunity, says Guest. According to recent studies, a daily probiotic can lessen cold symptoms and reduce time spent sick with respiratory illness. A recent meta-analysis showed that 3,451 subjects (athlete and non-athlete) likely benefited from probiotics, so what do you have to lose? Researchers have also speculated—but have yet to see enough research to validate—that probiotics are especially helpful to athletes by improving immune function, aiding in digestion, and even enhancing athletic performance in hot weather.

Vitamin D supplementation can increase your immunity—but refer to what we already talked about in Chapter 16: A larger dose isn't always better. Your skin and body can regulate when vitamin D is introduced naturally, but you lack the same control with supplements and, therefore, have an increased risk of overdosing, which can lead to calcium buildup (and nausea, loss of appetite, and general weakness). It's hard to overdose with food, but some supplements may put you over the line: The recommended dose is 600 IU, and it takes supplementing with 50,000 IUs a day of vitamin D for several months before toxicity levels become a concern.

## INJURY

If you're injured, and not simply sick, there are three targets to aid recovery. First, Guest says, focus on inflammation management (note that we're not advocating getting rid of inflammation altogether). Second, focus on immune support, and last, preserve muscle mass.

Regarding inflammation, you've likely heard in recent years that icing to decrease inflammation or taking nonsteroidal anti-inflammatory drugs (NSAIDs) to decrease swelling are both becoming more and more controversial. That's where nutrition can come in handy. Some inflammation is important to recovery, as it forces us to take time off to heal, but excessive inflammation can increase total tissue damage and slow down repair, Guest warns. "Respect the purpose of inflammation," she says. It happens for a reason, and while we can decrease it, we don't want to mask the body's natural healing process.

There are certain ways you can shift to more of an inflammation-fighting diet. First, cut back on certain fats. Trans fats, omega-6-rich vegetable oils, and saturated fat are, sadly, pro-inflammatory. In their place, increase your intake of monounsaturated fats and omega-3 fats, which are anti-inflammatory. And last, increase your vitamin D intake since it down-regulates the expression of inflammatory cytokines.

When injured, preserving muscle mass will likely be your greatest challenge—you didn't climb all those hills just to watch your quads shrivel while you nurse a bum knee, right? Healthy, inactive muscle decreases at a rate of 0.5 percent per day, and the first 1 to 2 weeks of off-the-bike time is when you experience the greatest loss. But the good news is that you can slow the muscle loss with vitamin C to increase collagen and vitamin D to promote skeletal muscle regeneration, explains Guest. And, of course, make sure you're getting enough protein, in the range of 15 to 20 grams at each meal. Even though you're not training, the protein will help reduce muscle loss. To get the best results, spread out your protein intake throughout the day, up to four to six times daily, and make sure you're getting the amino acid leucine (found in whey protein powder).

Being sick or injured is a bummer, but the best thing you can do is take time to recover before you throw yourself back into training. Don't risk a season for the sake of a week.

## YOUR FIVE TAKEAWAYS

1. Avoid getting sick: Start taking probiotics to improve gut health and immunity.

2. Stay hydrated and take in an adequate amount of carbs to decrease the risk of illness and to keep your system functioning properly if you are sick.

3. If sick or injured, increase your protein intake in order to speed up recovery and preserve muscle.

4. If injured, cut back on certain fats to decrease inflammation.

5. Taking a day off to recover from illness may save you a week off the bike later.

# CHAPTER EIGHTEEN

# THE FUTURE OF ATHLETE NUTRITION— SPORT GENOMICS

All cyclists aren't created equal, some are just genetically gifted. While you can work to improve what you're given, unfortunately, it takes more than grit and determination to propel you into the upper echelon of the competitive sports world. You may be able to win local races or hold the Strava title King of the Mountain on a tough climb, but the odds of making it as a top level Pro Tour rider are incredibly slim. You can thank your genes for that.

Nanci Guest, MSc, RD, CSCS, focuses primarily on how human genetics impact athletic development. She explains, "Human athletic performance is quite variable and highly complex. For example, two male power athletes of similar age, experience, and body composition who follow the same resistance-training program under close supervision. At the end of

8 weeks, one has gained nearly 5 pounds of muscle and the other has gained none. Why? Genes.

"When researchers examine the link between diet and disease, supplements and performance, or training methods and improved speed or power, why do the observed outcomes have such mixed results?" she asks. "Only over the last few years has this mystery started to unravel." Guest has dedicated her career to answering such questions.

After the complete sequencing of the human genome in 2003, the field of genetics took a front seat in scientific research, but the majority of research focused on illness and disease prevention. However, thousands of genes that are relevant to fitness and performance have been identified since the Human Genome Project decoded the 3 billion letter pairs that make up our DNA, and Guest is proudly part of this exciting development. "These range from genes affecting cardiovascular endurance, muscle power, and strength to genes related to pain intolerance, mental focus, recovery heart rate, body composition, blood pressure, and metabolic factors such as lactic acid clearance and energy utilization," she explains. "Along with the identification of exercise-related genetic characteristics, there is evidence that specific genetic profiles may be very responsive to a particular exercise regimen and nonresponsive to another. This means we should aim to reach our genetic potential by training what we're born with, while still considering the influence of environmental factors, such as coaching and access to training facilities."

This comes as no surprise to most coaches, who understand that individual athletes require different programs to be successful. "Strength and conditioning coaches have understood for years that there is a need to tailor workouts and training routines to each individual without knowing the genetics involved, but as the science emerges, we should be able to optimize individual training programs based on an athlete's genetic profile," Guest says.

"For example, over a decade ago, a variation in the angiotensin I-converting enzyme (ACE) gene became the first genetic element to be linked to human physical performance," Guest continues. "Although this gene has offered insight into an athlete's likelihood to be more successful at endurance sports versus power sports, there is still a lot of work to be done before we can predict future athletic success. In the meantime, we can clearly see associations between genes, muscle function, and exercise capacity. For instance, genes such as muscle fiber type (ACTN3), red blood cell production and function (EPOR; HBB) as well as mitochondrial numbers and activity (PGC-1a) and others, are all necessary to better understand the limits of our endurance capabilities and identify the areas that need more attention in order to achieve our full genetic potential."

## NUTRIGENOMICS

So how does nutrition factor in? Nutrigenomics is the study of how genes affect the way we absorb, metabolize, and utilize nutrients and how the interaction between genes and diet can influence our health and performance. "Genetic differences can affect how we respond to the foods, beverages, and supplements we consume, and how that ultimately influences our nutritional status, health, and ultimately performance," explains Guest. This is the reason why some people do well on high-fat diets, while others pack on weight quickly when they increase their fat intake. Genetic differences are also why certain athletes are better suited for ultra-endurance, and others struggle to take in enough fuel to power through a 2-hour race.

"Why individuals experience different performance outcomes or struggle with body composition although they consume similar diets and calories or have similar pre- and post-exercise nutrition strategies and comparable training protocols is an important question that has been on the minds of sport-science researchers and sport-nutrition experts for years," says Guest. "While it has long been suspected that genetics plays a critical role in determining how a person responds to foods and nutrients, only recently has research in the field of nutrigenomics demonstrated this. 'Eat according to your genes' takes personalized nutrition to a whole new level." Forget trial and error—now you can take your performance diet to a whole new level by aligning it with your DNA.

"Studies of gene–environment relationships have also shown that variations in genes involved in nutrient metabolism can affect our response to certain diets, such as our ability to better lose weight on a high-carb versus high-fat diet, along with different recommendations for protein intake," she adds. "Studies on the influence of genetic variants on dietary response patterns are paving the way for personalized approaches to fat loss."

Genes may also be responsible for the way in which supplements affect your diet. For some, supplements like caffeine are extremely useful, while for other athletes, caffeine may not have any positive effect. "There is dramatic variability in inter-individual response to any type of supplement or dietary interven-

tion," Guest explains. "For example, some people do not utilize vitamin C from the diet as efficiently as others and are at a greater risk of vitamin C deficiency. Vitamin C is a well-known antioxidant that aids in the ability to reduce exercise-induced oxidative damage, which translates into better recovery from training and greater resistance to fatigue. However, too much vitamin C can also be harmful to performance as it can interfere with the body's natural adaptation to training, so the more-is-better approach may prove to be just as harmful as a deficiency."

Nutrigenomics is still a relatively new field, and testing is somewhat expensive. "Sport genomics is still in the early phase, and more research is needed before the preliminary findings can be extended to mainstream practice in sport," explains Guest. "Although DNA profiling cannot detect or determine who will be a superior athlete, it can predict potential abilities and weaknesses associated with specific aspects of sports performance. Future research including genome-wide association studies; whole-genome sequencing; and epigenetic, transcriptomic, and proteomic profiling will allow a better understanding of genetic makeup and molecular physiology of the broad-spectrum of athletic capabilities."

The future is bright for additional research, and we may soon be incorporating many of these concepts into personalized training programs. "It is an exciting time in sport genomics as we begin to create the necessary tools to develop personalized programs that will allow sport-science professionals and practitioners to collaborate in a paradigm shift that will improve our ability to achieve optimal health, fitness, and athletic performance," Guest concludes. "Once personalized training and nutrition is integrated into routine practice, we can better predict efficacy of various training programs, diets, and ergogenic aids, as well as determine risks for injuries and nutrient deficiencies that affect health and performance. When it comes to athletic performance, the emerging science of sport genomics will be the competitive edge of our future."

Until then, the information in this book will set you on the right path. Remember, as Guest said earlier, the research that's already out there is more than enough to reach the competitive level, but our genes will eventually determine the best way to eke out additional marginal training gains for each of us, individually.

You have all of the proper tools to make your nutrition work for you—on and off the bike—regardless of whether you eat meat or choose a vegetarian diet, prefer to live gluten-free or love a slice of toast in the morning. Whatever diet you subscribe to, as long as it's healthy, whole-foods based, includes plenty of vegetables, and focuses on fueling your ride—before, during, and after—you'll be ready for any ride. With optimal nutrition tailored to your specific needs and preferences—and plenty of practice on and off the bike!—you will see improvement in your cycling performance and overall health.

So, what are you waiting for? Get on that bike and get moving!

# APPENDIX: TESTING

## GET YOUR WEIGHT RIGHT

One of the best ways you can prep for a winning season is by knowing what you're up against. Keeping yourself honest with a food diary is a great start, but taking regular body measurements creates an important advantage when interpreting the nutritional data you so diligently recorded.

To start, knowing yourself means having a good idea of where you are in relation to your ideal body weight. This may mean shelling out big bucks for a DEXA (duel-energy x-ray absorptiometry) scan to get a perfect representation of your body-fat percentage or buying an impedance scale or just stepping on your normal bathroom scale. Regardless of the method, if weight and/or body mass is one of the things you're focusing on, knowledge is certainly power.

Once you know your current weight and have a grasp of your goal or optimal racing weight, it's time to look at other tests.

## BASIC BLOOD PANELS

Heading to your doctor for a regular physical is a smart move no matter who you are, but if you're an athlete, it's even more important. Ask your doctor to order a blood test to see if there are any vitamins or minerals that you may be deficient in. At the very least, test for the major vitamins and minerals, including vitamin D, iron, and the B vitamins. Blood panels are even more important for vegan and vegetarian athletes, who run a greater risk of having a nutrient deficiency.

"You should absolutely do a basic panel," says Nanci Guest, MSc, RD, CSCS. "The only way to know your true status is by doing the blood work."

Not all vitamins and minerals should be taken in high doses, so if you're not deficient, your body won't appreciate the overload. "You don't want to start taking iron or high-dosing vitamin D if you don't know where you're at," Guest adds. "And you don't want to fool around with iron, because it can be toxic. So you shouldn't supplement until you're sure."

It's not just about your overall health: Your training can also be impacted by low—or high—levels of a particular vitamin or mineral. "Blood testing is important because it gives you a chance to find out if you're lower or higher in certain things like iron or vitamin C," says Guest. "If you are naturally high in one, then supplementing may actually blunt adaptation and hurt training, and conversely, if you're low in one of the essential vitamins or minerals, you may be hit with things like fatigue and blunted performance."

## METABOLIC TESTING

If you're desperate to shed those last couple pounds and haven't had any success with diet and exercise, consider a metabolic test. "You can go in and get metabolic testing to see if you're a higher carb or fat burner so you know how to manipulate your diet, but that's getting really extreme," says Guest.

For those of you who aren't quite as numbers driven, don't worry about metabolic testing. "Those online calculators that tell you how much you're burning and what your metabolic rate is are fine," says Guest.

Additionally, metabolic rate isn't all it's cracked up to be, no matter how high-tech the lab is. "What people need to be aware of is that the metabolic rate is going to be a bit higher if you're a bit leaner, because you're going to have more metabolically active tissue with muscle," she adds. "One thing to keep in mind, too, is that someone dieting will see that base drop. Someone who's been dieting and reducing calories may have adapted to less. There are so many variables."

Remember that just because a test shows that you burn carbohydrates better than fat is not an excuse to start eating bread like it's going out of style, even after you hit your goal weight. Nutrient density is still king when it comes to proper food choice.

## CHECK YOUR HYDRATION

You now know that drinking according to thirst isn't the most accurate way to avoid dehydration or overhydration on the bike (see Chapter 10). But how do you know if you're drinking enough? It's time to get up close and personal with your pee and do some easy at-home testing.

Stacy Sims, MSc, PhD, suggests Rapid Response Urinalysis Reagent Test Strips (10 Parameter). "You can buy them online and do it yourself," she explains. "You want to be looking at your specific urine gravity (SG) and trying to maintain it, primarily."

While you don't have to test yourself every time you go on a ride, it can be a great way to determine how much you should be drinking—don't forget, a bottle per hour is just a starting point.

"You should start your activity around 1.015 or 1.020 SG and at the end of training, you shouldn't be in the 1.030 range, you want to be in the 1.025," says Dr. Sims. "That shows you're maintaining a good amount of body fluid—you might be a bit passively dehydrated but that's okay, because you can recover from that. But if you go over the edge of 1.030 or above, it takes a good amount of time to come back from that."

You can also check a few other measurements on the same strip, explains Dr. Sims. For leukocytes (white blood cells), the strip should stay the same color. If it turns purple, that's an indication that you have leukocytes in your system, which means you aren't properly recovered.

The same inadequate recovery will also show up on the protein section of the strip. According to Dr. Sims, green is normal within a few hours after exercise, but if you're seeing it the morning after a workout, you need more time to recover.

Last, check your ketones color. A positive test result indicates poor carbohydrate metabolization. If you're training, this may indicate that you aren't fueling enough, and you may want to eat more.

Again, you don't need to test your urine on a constant basis, but it's a great tool to establish baselines for hydration and even worth testing in different climates, like riding outside in the winter versus riding in the summer when you sweat more. And check in on the other measurements occasionally. If you feel run-down and are possibly overtraining, consider checking the other metrics for insight to your current body function in relation to your performance.

## GENETIC TESTING

If you love testing and data, consider going all out and getting a genetic test done. Most of the things we've talked about in this book are heavily influenced by our genes, and while we can manipulate our diets to make us into lean, mean racing machines, some of us will always be more gifted riders, thanks to our genes.

Even if it's not fair, at least you can find out what works best for you.

"I think there's going to be a paradigm shift, and we're going to start looking at raw data and at the outliers in studies, and trying to see if there's a genetic reason that they are the outliers," says Guest. "So, for example, we may start finding out which gene type beetroot juice is most effective for when it comes to performance."

If you want the whole picture, a nutrigenomics test[3] can be pretty interesting. It's more in-depth than the short-lived blood-type diet test, as it looks at fat and analyzes carbohydrate metabolism, lactose intolerance, and caffeine and vitamin D metabolism. The test, which is similar to a metabolic test but much more in-depth, can offer insight into how you should structure your macronutrient needs to best fuel your training.

Look for the right genetic test; one that focuses on nutrition rather than other health factors. Most genetic tests can be purchased online as units and the whole process—spitting in a vial and sealing it for delivery—takes a few seconds. Then, in a few weeks, you should have some interesting data to work with, like how your body responds to fat and protein, genes associated with obesity, and information on your genotype as an athlete.

[3] lifegenetics.net/faq/nutrigenomics/

# BIBLIOGRAPHY

## Introduction

M. Rosenbaum and R. L. Leibel, "Adaptive Thermogenesis in Humans," *International Journal of Obesity* 34 (2010): S47–55.

## Chapter One: Why Does It Matter?

Cynthia L. Curl, Shirley A. A. Beresford, Richard A. Fenske, Annette L. Fitzpatrick, Chensheng Lu, Jennifer A. Nettleton, and Joel D. Kaufman, "Estimating Pesticide Exposure from Dietary Intake and Organic Food Choices: The Multi-Ethnic Study of Atherosclerosis (MESA)," *Environmental Health Perspectives* 123, no. 5 (May 2015): 475–83; doi: 10.1289/ehp.1408197.

Ron J. Maughan and Susan M. Shirreffs, "IOC Consensus Conference on Nutrition in Sport, 25–27 October 2010, International Olympic Committee, Lausanne, Switzerland," *Journal of Sports Sciences* 29, Suppl 1 (2011): S1.

## Chapter Two: Fat

P. J. Cox and K. Clarke, "Acute Nutritional Ketosis: Implications for Exercise Performance and Metabolism," *Extreme Physiology and Medicine* 3 (October 29, 2014): 17.

J. W. Helge, "Adaptation to a Fat-Rich Diet: Effects on Endurance Performance in Humans," *Sports Medicine* 30, no. 5 (November 2000): 347–57.

G. Michas, R. Micha, and A. Zampelas, "Dietary Fats and Cardiovascular Disease: Putting Together the Pieces of a Complicated Puzzle," *Atherosclerosis* 234, no. 2 (June 2014): 320–28.

U. Schwab, L. Lauritzen, T. Tholstrup, T. Haldorssoni, U. Riserus, M. Uusitupa, and W. Becker, "Effect of the Amount and Type of Dietary Fat on Cardiometabolic Risk Factors and Risk of Developing Type 2 Diabetes, Cardiovascular Diseases, and Cancer: A Systematic Review," *Food and Nutrition Research* 58 (July 2014): 58. 10.3402/fnr.v58.25145. PMC. Web. 12 Sept. 2015.

L. L. Spriet, "New Insights into the Interaction of Carbohydrate and Fat Metabolism during Exercise," *Sports Medicine* 44, Suppl 1 (May 2014): S87–96.

Li Wang, Peter L. Bordi, Jennifer A. Fleming, Alison M. Hill, and Penny M. Kris-Etherton, "Effect of a Moderate Fat Diet with and without Avocados on Lipoprotein Particle Number, Size, and Subclasses in Overweight and Obese Adults: A Randomized, Controlled Trial," *Journal of the American Heart Association* 4, no. 1 (January 2015): 1–14; doi: 10.1161/JAHA.114.001355.

## Chapter Three: Protein

G. Biolo, K. D. Tipton, S. Klein, and R. R. Wolfe, "An Abundant Supply of Amino Acids Enhances the Metabolic Effect of Exercise on Muscle Protein," *American Journal of Physiology* 273, (1997): E122–29.

Bill Campbell, Richard B Kreider, Tim Ziegenfuss, Paul La Bounty, Mike Roberts, Darren Burke, Jamie Landis, Hector Lopez, and Jose Antonio, "International Society of Sports Nutrition Position Stand: Protein and Exercise," *Journal of the International Society of Sports Nutrition* 8. Accessed January 26, 2015.

S. J. Crozier, S. R. Kimball, S. W. Emmert, J. C. Anthony, and L. S. Jefferson, "Oral Leucine Administration Stimulates Protein Synthesis in Rat Skeletal Muscle," *Journal of Nutrition* 135, (2005): 376–82.

D. Cuthbertson, K. Smith, J. Babraj, G. Leese, T. Waddell, P. Atherton, H. Wackerhage, P. M. Taylor, and M. J. Rennie, "Anabolic Signaling Deficits Underlie Amino Acid Resistance of Wasting, Aging Muscle," *FASEB Journal* 19, (2005): 422–24.

S. Phillips, "Dietary Protein Requirements and Adaptive Advantages in Athletes," *British Journal of Nutrition* 108, (2012): S158–67.

———, "The Importance of Dietary Protein in Resistance Exercise-Induced Adaption: All Proteins are not Created Equal," Exercise Metabolism Research Group, McMaster Univ. Webinar, October, 18 2012.

A. Philp, D. L. Hamilton, and K. Baar, "Signals Mediating Skeletal Muscle Remodeling by Resistance Exercise: PI3-Kinase Independent Activation of mTORC1," *Journal of Applied Physiology* 110, (2011): 561–68.

Jichun Yang, Yujing Chi, Brant R. Burkhardt, Youfei Guan, and Bryan A. Wolf, "Leucine Metabolism in Regulation of Insulin Secretion from Pancreatic Beta Cells," *Nutrition Reviews* 68, no. 5 (May 2010): 270–79.

## Chapter Four: Carbohydrates

Jessica R. Biesiekierski, Simone L. Peters, Evan D. Newnham, Ourania Rosella, Jane G. Muir, and Peter R. Gibson, "No Effects of Gluten in Patients with Self-Reported Non-Celiac Gluten Sensitivity after Dietary Reduction of Fermentable, Poorly Absorbed, Short-Chain Carbohydrates," *Gastroenterology* 145, no. 2 (2013): 320–28.

J. P. Cappon, "Acute Effects of High-Fat and High-Glucose Meals on the Growth Hormone Response to Exercise," *Journal of Clinical Endocrinology and Metabolism* 76, no. 6 (1993): 1418–22.

D. Dreher and A. F. Junod, "Role of Oxygen-Free Radicals in Cancer Development," *European Journal of Cancer* 32, no. 1 (1996): 30–38.

Peter Gibson and Susan Shepard, "Evidence-Based Dietary Management of Functional Gastrointestinal Symptoms: The FODMAP Approach," *Journal of Gastroenterology and Hepatology* 25, no. 2 (February 2010): 252–58.

M. Ristow, K. Zarse, A. Oberbach, N. Kloting, M. Birringer, M. Kiehntopf, M. Stumvoll, C. R. Kahn, and M. Bluher, "Antioxidants Prevent Health-Promoting Effects of Physical Exercise in Humans," *Proceedings of the National Academy of Sciences* 106, no. 21 (2009): 8665–70.

Joanne L. Slavin, "Dietary Fiber and Body Weight," *Nutrition* 21, no. 3 (2005): 411–18.

## Chapter Five: Breakfast

A. W. Brown, M. M. Bohan Brown, and D. B. Allison, "Belief beyond the Evidence: Using the Proposed Effect of Breakfast on Obesity to Show Two Practices That Distort Scientific Evidence," *American Journal of Clinical Nutrition* 98, no. 5 (November 2013): 1298–1308.

## Chapter Seven: Snacks

Asker E. Jeukendrup, "Nutrition for Endurance Sports: Marathon, Triathlon, and Road Cycling," *Journal of Sport Sciences* 29, Suppl 1 (2011): S91–99.

M. J. Ormsbee, C. W. Back, and D. A. Baur, "Pre-Exercise Nutrition: The Role of Macronutrients, Modified Starches, and Supplements on Metabolism and Endurance Performance," *Nutrients* 6, no. 5 (April 29, 2014): 1782–1808.

## Chapter Eight: Dinner

M. E. Clegg, V. Ranawana, A. Shafat, and C. J. Henry, "Soups Increase Satiety through Delayed Gastric Emptying yet Increased Glycaemic Response," *European Journal of Clinical Nutrition* 67, no. 1 (January 2013): 8–11.

E. A. Dennis, A. L. Dengo, D. L. Comber, et al., "Water Consumption Increases Weight Loss During a Hypocaloric Diet Intervention in Middle-Aged and Older Adults," *Obesity* 18, no. 2 (2010): 300–307.

## Chapter Nine: Everything in Moderation

M. J. Barnes, T. Mundel, and S. R. Stannard, "The Effects of Acute Alcohol Consumption and Eccentric Muscle Damage on Neuromuscular

Function," *Applied Physiology, Nutrition, and Metabolism* 37, no. 1 (2011): 63–71.

S. N. Cheuvront and R. W. Kenefick, "Dehydration: Physiology, Assessment, and Performance Effects," *Comprehensive Physiology* 4, no. 1 (January 2014): 257–85.

P. Greiffenstein, C. V. Stouwe, et al., "Alcohol-Binge Prior to Trauma-Hemorrhage Results in Sustained Derangement of Host Inflammatory Responses during Recovery," *Alcoholism: Clinical and Experimental Research* 31, no. 4 (2007): 704–15.

Alistair P. Murphy, Alanna E. Snape, Geoffrey M. Minett, Melissa Skein, and Rob Duffield, "The Effect of Post-Match Alcohol Ingestion on Recovery from Competitive Rugby League Matches," *Journal of Strength and Conditioning Research* 27, no. 5 (2013): 1304–12.

C. Prentice, S. R. Stannard, and M. J. Barnes, "The Effects of Binge Drinking Behaviour on Recovery and Performance after a Rugby Match," *Journal of Science and Medicine in Sport* 17, no. 2 (2013): 244–48.

T. Roehrs, J. Yoon, and T. Roth, "Nocturnal and Next-Day Effects of Ethanol and Basal Level of Sleepiness," *Human Psychopharmacology: Clinical and Experimental* 6, no. 4 (1991): 307–11.

T. L. Rupp, C. Acebo, and M. A. Carskadon, "Evening Alcohol Suppresses Salivary Melatonin in Young Adults," *Chronobiology International* 24, no. 3 (2007): 463–70.

Susan M. Shirreffs and Ronald J. Maughan, "The Effect of Alcohol on Athletic Performance," *Current Sports Medicine Reports* 5, no. 4 (2006): 192–96.

———, "Restoration of Fluid Balance after Exercise-Induced Dehydration: Effects of Alcohol Consumption," *Journal of Applied Physiology* 83, no. 4 (1997): 1152–58.

G. Szabo, "Consequences of Alcohol Consumption on Host Defence," *Alcohol* 34, no.6 (1999): 830–41.

M. R. Yeomans, "Alcohol, Appetite, and Energy Balance: Is Alcohol Intake a Risk Factor for Obesity?" *Physiology and Behavior* 100, no. 1 (April 26, 2010): 82–89.

X. J. Zhao, L. Marrero, K. Song, et al., "Acute Alcohol Inhibits TNF-alpha Processing in Human Monocytes by Inhibiting TNF/TNF-alpha-Converting Enzyme Interactions in the Cell Membrane," *Journal of Immunology* 170, no. 6 (2003): 2923–31.

## Part Three: Your Ride

H. Skolnik and A. Chernus, *Nutrient Timing for Peak Performance: The Right Food, the Right Time, the Right Results* (Champaign, IL: Human Kinetics, 2010).

## Chapter Ten: In-Exercise Hydration

J. R. Berning and S. N. Steen, *Nutrition for Sport and Exercise*, Second Edition (Sudbury, MA: Jones and Bartlett Publishers, 2006).

C. Capitan, J. D. Adams, L. Summers, E. C. Johnson, and S. A. Kavouras, "Hydration Habits During a Recreational Mountain Bike Race," *International Journal of Exercise Science*: Conference Proceedings: Vol. 11: Issue 2, Article 8 (2014).

M. C. Devries, M. J. Hamadeh, S. M. Phillips, et al., "Menstrual Cycle Phase and Sex Influence Muscle Glycogen Utilization and Glucose Turnover during Moderate-Intensity Endurance Exercise," *American Journal of Physiology—Regulatory, Integrative and Comparative Physiology* 291, no. 4 (2006): R1120–28.

W. Latzka and S. Montain, "Water and Electrolyte Requirements for Exercise," *Clinics in Sports Medicine* 18, no. 3 (1999): 513–24.

Michael R. Simpson and Tom Howard, "ACSM Information on Selecting and Effectively Using Hydration for Fitness," acsm.org/docs/brochures/selecting-and-effectively-using-hydration-for-fitness.pdf. Accessed February 1, 2015.

S. T. Sims, N. J. Rehrer, M. L. Bell, and J. D. Cotter, "Endogenous and Exogenous Female Sex Hormones and Renal Electrolyte Handling: Effects of an Acute Sodium Load on Plasma Volume at Rest," *Journal of Applied Physiology* 105, no. 1 (2008): 121–27.

———, "Preexercise Sodium Loading Aids Fluid Balance and Endurance for Women Exercising in the Heat," *Journal of Applied Physiology* 103, no. 2 (2007): 534–41.

P. B. Wilson and S. J. Ingraham, "Glucose-Fructose Likely Improves Gastrointestinal Comfort and Endurance Running Performance Relative to Glucose-Only," *Scandinavian Journal of Medicine and Science in Sports*. doi: 10.1111/sms.12386.

## Chapter Eleven: In-Exercise Food

J. Achten, "Higher Dietary Carbohydrate Content during Intensified Running Training Results in Better Maintenance of Performance and Mood State," *Journal of Applied Physiology* 96, no. 4 (2004): 1331–40.

Keith Baar, "Nutrition and the Adaptation to Endurance Training," *Sports Medicine* 44, no. 1 (2014): 5–12.

K. Baar, et al., "Adaptations of Skeletal Muscle to Exercise: Rapid Increase in the Transcriptional Coactivator PGC-1," *FASEB Journal* 16, no. 14 (2002): 1879.

Michael Gleeson, "Immune Function in Sport and Exercise," *Journal of Applied Physiology* 103, no. 2 (2007): 693–99.

E. R. Goldstein, T. Ziegenfuss, D. Kalman, et al., "International Society of Sports Nutrition Position Stand: Caffeine and Performance," *Journal of the International Society of Sports Nutrition* 7, no. 5 (2010): 1–15.

Carl J. Hulston, Michelle C. Venables, Chris H. Mann, Cara Martin, Andrew Philp, Keith Baar, and Asker E. Jeukendrup, "Training with Low Muscle Glycogen Enhances Fat Metabolism in Well-Trained Cyclists," *Medicine and Science in Sports and Exercise* 42, no. 11 (2010): 2046–55.

Asker Jeukendrup, "A Step towards Personalized Sports Nutrition," *Sports Medicine* 44, Suppl. 1 (2014): S25–33.

J. Lin, et al., "Metabolic control through the PGC-1 family of transcription coactivators." *Cell Metabolism* 1, no. 6 (2005): 361-70.

T. T. Peternelj and J. S. Coombes, "Antioxidant Supplementation during Exercise Training: Beneficial or Detrimental?" *Sports Medicine* 41, no. 12 (December 1, 2011): 1043–69.

B. J. Schoenfeld, et al., "Body Composition Changes Associated with Fasted versus Non-Fasted Aerobic Exercise," *Journal of the International Society of Sports Nutrition* 11 (2014): 54.

Orestis-Konstantinos Tsintzas, Clyde Williams, Wendy Wilson, and Jackie Burrin, "Influence of Carbohydrate Supplementation Early in Exercise on Endurance Running Capacity," *Medicine and Science in Sports and Exercise* 28, no. 11 (1996): 1373–79.

## Chapter Twelve: In-Race Food

E. P. de Oliveira, R. C. Burini, A. Jeukendrup, "Gastrointestinal Complaints during Exercise: Prevalence, Etiology, and Nutritional Recommendations," *Sports Medicine* 44, Suppl. 1 (2014): S79–85.

K. van Wijck, K. Lenaerts, L. J. van Loon, W. H. Peters, W. A. Buurman, and C. H. Dejong, "Exercise-Induced Splanchnic Hypoperfusion Results in Gut Dysfunction in Healthy Men," *PLOS One* 6, no. 7 (2011): 1–9. doi: 10.1371/journal.pone.0022366. Epub 2011 Jul 21.

Kim van Wijck, Kaatje Lenaerts, Annemarie A. van Bijnen, Bas Boonen, Luc J. C. van Loon, Cornelis H. C. Dejong, and Wim A. Buurman, "Aggravation of Exercise-Induced Intestinal Injury by Ibuprofen in Athletes," *Medicine and Science in Sports and Exercise* 44, no. 12 (2012): 2257–62.

## Chapter Thirteen: Post-Ride Food

Sarah R. Jackman, Oliver C. Witard, Asker E. Jeukendrup, and Kevin D. Tipton, "Branched-Chain Amino Acid Ingestion Can Ameliorate Soreness from Eccentric Exercise," *Medicine and Science in Sports and Exercise* 42, no. 5 (2009): 962–70.

## Chapter Fourteen: Weight Loss

M. L. Butryn, S. Phelan, J. O. Hill, and R. R. Wing, "Consistent Self-Monitoring of Weight: A Key Component of Successful Weight-Loss Maintenance," *Obesity* 15, no. 12 (2007): 3091–96. doi: 10.1038/oby.2007.368

Elina E. Helander, Anna-Leena Vuorinen, Brian Wansink, and Ilkka K. J. Korhonen, "Are Breaks in Daily Self-Weighing Associated with Weight Gain?" *PLOS One* 9, no. 11 (2014): 1–6 DOI: 10.1371/journal.pone.0113164.

J. Alfredo Martinez, "Personalized Weight-Loss Strategies—The Role of Macronutrient Distribution," *Nature Reviews Endocrinology* 10 (2014): 749-60.

D. S. Soni, J. D. Wagganer, and M. M. Abdul, "Impact of Professional Nutrition Program on a Female Cross Country Athlete: Case Study," *International Journal of Exercise Science:* Conference Proceedings: Vol. 11: Issue 2, Article 58 (2014).

## Chapter Fifteen: Stress, Food Intolerance, and the Cyclist

G. Addolorato, "Anxiety and Depression: A Common Feature of Health Care Seeking Patients with Irritable Bowel Syndrome and Food Allergy," *Hepato-Gastroenterology* 45, no. 23 (1998): 1559–64.

Elissa S. Epel, Bruce McEwen, Teresa Seeman, Karen Matthews, Grace Castellazzo, Kelly D. Brownell, Jennifer Bell, and Jeannette R. Ickovics, "Stress and Body Shape: Stress-Induced Cortisol Secretion Is Consistently Greater among Women with Central Fat," *Psychosomatic Medicine* 62, no. 5 (September/October 2000): 623–32.

Investigación y Desarrollo. "Poor Sleep Causes Weight Gain, Susceptibility to Diabetes," *Science Daily* 3 (2015). sciencedaily.com/releases/2015/01/150103072440.htm. Accessed January 5, 2015.

Jan Machal, "Chronobiology, Sleep Disturbances, and Food Intake Disorders," *Appetite: Regulation, Use of Stimulants and Cultural and Biological Influences.*

Ed. Julie Bienertova-Vasku (Hauppauge, NY: Nova Science, 2014). 15-44. Print.

Matthew D. Milewski, David L. Skaggs, Gregory A. Bishop, J. Lee Pace, David A. Ibrahim, Tishya A. L. Wren, and Audrius Barzdukas, "Chronic Lack of Sleep Is Associated with Increased Sports Injuries in Adolescent Athletes," *Journal of Pediatric Orthopaedics* 34, no. 2 (2014): 129–33.

P. M. Peeke and G. P. Chrousos, "Hypercortisolism and Obesity," *Annals of the New York Academy of Sciences* 771, (December 29, 1995): 665–76.

Piero Vernia, Mauro Di Camillo, Tiziana Foglietta, Veronica E. Avallone, and Aurora De Carolis, "Diagnosis of Lactose Intolerance and the 'Nocebo' Effect: The Role of Negative Expectations," *Digestive and Liver Disease* 42, no. 9 (2010): 616–19.

## Chapter Sixteen: Supplements

Thomas W. Buford, Richard B Kreider, Jeffrey R. Stout, Mike Greenwood, Bill Campbell, Marie Spano, Tim Ziegenfuss, Hector Lopez, Jamie Landis, and Jose Antonio, "International Society of Sports Nutrition Position Stand: Creatine Supplementation and Exercise," *Journal of the International Society of Sports Nutrition* 6. Accessed January 26, 2015.

Center for Science in the Public Interest, "Caffeine Content of Food and Drugs," November 1, 2014. Accessed March 17, 2015. cspinet.org/new/cafchart.htm.

K. De Pauw, B. Roelands, K. Knaepen, M. Polfliet, J. Stiens, R. Meeusen, "Effects of Caffeine and Maltodextrin Mouth Rinsing on P300, Brain Imaging and Cognitive Performance," *Journal of Applied Physiology* 118, no. 6 (2015): 776–82. jap .01050.2014. doi: 10.1152/japplphysiol .01050. 2014.

B. Desbrow, C. Biddulph, B. Devlin, G. D. Grant, S. Anoopkumar-Dukie, M. D. Leveritt, "The Effects of Different Doses of Caffeine on Endurance Cycling Time Trial Performance," *Journal of Sports Sciences* 30, No. 2 (2012): 115–20.

M. S. Ganio et al., "Effect of Caffeine on Sport-Specific Endurance Performance: A Systematic Review," *Journal of Strength and Conditioning Research* 23, no. 1 (2009): 315–24.

R. C. Gliottoni et al., "Effect of Caffeine on Quadricep Pain during Acute Cycling Exercises in Low versus High Caffeine Consumers," *International Journal of Sport Nutrition and Exercise Metabolism* 19 (2009): 150–61.

E. R. Goldstein, T. Ziegenfuss, D. Kalman et al., "International Society of Sports Nutrition Position Stand: Caffeine and Performance," *Journal of the International Society of Sports Nutrition* 7 (2010): 5. doi: 10.1186/1550-2783-7-5.

A. B. Hodgson, R. K. Randell, and A. E. Jeukendrup, "The Metabolic and Performance Effects of Caffeine Compared to Coffee during Endurance Exercise," *PLOS One* 8, No. 4 (2013): 1–10.

A. P. S. Hungin, C. Mulligan, B. Pot, et al., "Systematic Review: Probiotics in the Management of Lower Gastrointestinal Symptoms in Clinical Practice—An Evidence-Based International Guide," *Alimentary Pharmacology and Therapeutics* 38, no. 8 (2013): 864–86. doi: 10.1111/apt.12460.

Institute of Medicine (IOM), *Dietary Reference Intakes for Calcium and Vitamin D* (Washington, DC: National Academies Press, 2011).

E. Larson-Meyer, "Vitamin D Supplementation in Athletes," *Nestle Nutrition Institute Workshop Series* 75 (2013): 109–21. doi: 10.1159/000345827. Epub 2013 Apr 16. PubMed PMID: 23765355.

T. T. Peternelj and J. S. Coombes, "Antioxidant Supplementation during Exercise Training: Beneficial or Detrimental?" *Sports Medicine* 41, no. 12 (December 1, 2011): 1043–69.

T. L. Skinner, D. G. Jenkins, J. S. Coombes, D. R. Taaffe, and M. D. Leveritt, "Dose Response of Caffeine on 2000-m Rowing Performance," *Medicine and Science in Sports and Exercise* 42, no. 3 (2010): 571–76.

L. V. Thomas, T. Ockhuizen, and K. Suzuki, "Exploring the Influence of the Gut Microbiota and Probiotics on Health: A Symposium Report," *British Journal of Nutrition* 112, Suppl. 1 (2014): S1–18.

P. R. Von Hurst and K. L. Beck, "Vitamin D and Skeletal Muscle Function in Athletes," *Current Opinion in Clinical Nutrition and Metabolic Care* 17, no. 6 (November 2014): 539–45.

## Chapter Seventeen: Immunity and the Cyclist

Claudia Buitrago, Verónica Gonzalez Pardo, and Ricardo Boland, "Role of VDR in 1α,25-dihydroxyvitamin D3-Dependent Non-Genomic Activation of MAPKs, Src and Akt in Skeletal Muscle Cells," *The Journal of Steroid Biochemistry and Molecular Biology* 136 (2013): 125–30.

Q. Han, Z. Lu, B. R. Dong, C. Q. Huang, and T. Wu, "Probiotics for Preventing Acute Upper Respiratory Tract Infections," *Cochrane Database System Review* 9 (September 7, 2011): CD006895. doi: 10.1002/14651858.CD006895.pub2.

D. J. Owens, W. D. Fraser, and G. L. Close, "Vitamin D and the Athlete: Emerging Insights," *European Journal of Sport Science* 15, no. 1 (2015): 73–84. doi: 10.1080/17461391.2014.944223.

Benjamin T. Wall, James P. Morton, and Luc J. C. Van Loon, "Strategies to Maintain Skeletal Muscle Mass in the Injured Athlete: Nutritional Considerations and Exercise Mimetics," *European Journal of Sport Science* 15, no. 1 (2014): 53–62.

N. P. Walsh, M. Gleeson, R. J. Shephard, M. Gleeson, J. A. Woods, N. C. Bishop, M. Fleshner, C. Green, B. K. Pedersen, L. Hoffman-Goetz, C. J. Rogers, H. Northoff, A. Abbasi, and P. Simon, "Position Statement. Part One: Immune Function and Exercise," *Exercise Immunology Review* 17 (2011): 6–63.

## Chapter Eighteen: The Future of Athlete Nutrition—Sport Genomics

T. A. Astorino et al., "Increases in Cycling Performance in Response to Caffeine Ingestion Are Repeatable," *Nutrition Research* 32, no. 2 (2012): 78–84.

J. T. Finnoff, E. J. Jelsing, and J. Smith, "Biomarkers, Genetics, and Risk Factors for Concussion," *Physical Medicine and Rehabilitation* 3, No. 10 Suppl. 2 (October 2011): S452-59.

N. T. Jenkins et al., "Ergogenic Effects of Low Doses of Caffeine on Cycling Performance," *International Journal of Sport Nutrition and Exercise Metabolism* 18, no. 3 (2008): 328–42.

M. Kambouris, F. Ntalouka, G. Ziogas, and N. Maffulli, "Predictive Genomics DNA Profiling for Athletic Performance," *Recent Patents on DNA and Gene Sequences* 6, no. 3 (2012): 229–39.

J. A. Martinez, S. Navas-Carretero, W. H. Saris, and A. Astrup, "Personalized Weight-Loss Strategies—The Role of Macronutrient Distribution," *Natural Reviews Endocrinology* 10, no. 12 (December 2014): 749–60.

H. E. Montgomery et al., "Human Gene for Physical Performance," *Nature* 393, no. 6682 (May 21, 1998): 221–22.

S. Powers et al., "Antioxidant and Vitamin D Supplements for Athletes: Sense or Nonsense?" *Journal of Sports Sciences* 29, Suppl. 1 (2011): S47–55.

M. Ristow et al., "Antioxidants Prevent Health-Promoting Effects of Physical Exercise in Humans," *Proceedings of the National Academy of Sciences USA* 106, no. 21 (May 2009): 8665–70.

B. Roelands et al., "No Effect of Caffeine on Exercise Performance in High Ambient Temperature," *European Journal of Applied Physiology* 111, no. 12 (2011): 3089–95.

C. J. Saunders, "Investigation of Variants within the COL27A1 and TNC Genes and Achilles Tendinopathy in Two Populations," *Journal of Orthopaedic Research* 31, no. 4 (April 2013): 632–37.

## Appendix: Testing

Elina E. Helander, Anna-Leena Vuorinen, Brian Wansink, and Ilkka K. J. Korhonen, "Are Breaks in Daily Self-Weighing Associated with Weight Gain?" *PLOS One* 9, no. 11 (2014): e113164 doi: 10.1371 /journal.pone.0113164

# ACKNOWLEDGMENTS

I'd like to thank all of the awesome experts and pros who took time out of their lives to help me put this book together. As I said throughout, I'm not an all-knowing nutrition guru, I'm just sharing the wisdom that so many pros and nutritionists have been subscribing to in order to be in top performance shape. But I'd especially like to thank Nanci Guest, who, in addition to being the primary expert in this book, has become a great friend in the process. I couldn't have written it without her, and her expertise has been invaluable.

Because this is the only time I get to give acceptance-speech-style thank-yous, I'm taking full advantage. The experts and professional racers who offered their knowledge and experience for this book made writing it feel like fun: Chatting with Ted King about maple syrup, joking with Georgia Gould about cupcakes, and finally getting my hands on Katie Compton's cookie recipe made researching feel more like gossiping with friends. And the experts were just as fun!

It takes a village to write a book, and the staff over at *Bicycling* magazine has been equally helpful, doling out advice, being supportive, and—with so many amazing writers and cyclists all in the same place—providing me with the motivation to love every single word I write about cycling. And, like every good acceptance speech, I'd like to thank my parents for putting up with my weird schedule and travel, including plenty of drop-in writing weekends.

# INDEX

Boldface page references indicate photographs and captions. Underscored references indicate boxed text or tables.

Takeaways, Your Five *(cont.)*
post-ride food, 143
protein, 34
sleep, 171
snacks, 71
stress, 171
supplements, 181
weight loss, 163
Tests
blood, 191–92
body weight, 191
doping, 173, 174, 179
genetic, 193
hydration, 192–93
metabolic, 192
vitamin/mineral
deficiencies, 175
Three R's of recovery, 139
Tomatoes
Guacamole, 22
Tayler Wiles's Herb-Filled
Salad with Quinoa,
Cherry Tomatoes, and
Almonds, 62
Tayler Wiles's Quinoa,
Bean, and Squash
Veggie Burgers, 80
Track cycling bike body, 6–7
Training. *See also* Endurance
training
aerobic/anaerobic capacity
and, 128
antioxidant supplements
and, 14
breakfast and, 51–52, 56–59
caloric requirements and,
112–13
carbohydrates and, 9, 30,
36–38, 44–45, 49, **49**,
124

chocolate and, 86–88
digestive problems and,
avoiding, 132–33
dinner and, 73–74
excessive, 161, 183
fasted state, 123–28, 127,
140, 178
fats and, 9, 23, 26, 49, **49**
food intolerances and, 167–
71, 168–69
gains in, visible, 124
genetics and, 188
glycogen stores and, 117
illness and, 183–85
individual needs and, 188
injury and, 183–86
intervals and, hard, 134
muscle soreness and, 128
nutrition and, ix–xii, **x**, 15,
95
off-season and, 91–92,
**157**
protein and, 9, 49, **49**
recovery after hard, 140
as science experiment, 2
sleep and, 165–66
snacks and, 69
strength, 31
stress and, 165
weight loss and, 118,
148–49
Trans fats, ix, 17, 23–24, 26
Travel to race, 136–37
Treats. *See* Snacks

## U

U.S. Department of
Agriculture (USDA),
35

## V

Vegan diet
breakfast, 54
dinner, 78–79, 81
fiber and, 39
iron deficiency and, 175
personal experiences with,
ix–x, 12–13
protein and, 28
supplements and, 174, 175
Vegetables. *See also specific
type*
cooking tips, 66
fresh, 39
as good carbohydrates, 38
organic, 42–43
pesticides and, 43, 56
pre-cut, 66
washing, 56
Vitamin, C, 186, 189
Vitamin D and vitamin D
deficiency, 176, 178,
185–86, 189, 191
Vitamin/mineral deficiencies
tests, 175
Vitamins. *See specific type*

## W

WADA, 174, 179
Washing fruits and
vegetables, 56
Water intake. *See* Hydration
Weather and hydration, 101–
2, 109, 193
Weighing in, 148, 149
Weight gain
alcohol and, 86
basal metabolic rate and, 9

# ABOUT THE AUTHORS

**Molly Hurford** is a writer-at-large for *Bicycling* magazine and has been in love with the science of cycling nutrition since she first started racing triathlons in college. From triathlons, she discovered that what she really loved was the bike and shifted to focusing on racing cyclocross and on the road. A few years later, she's still racing and rides as much as is humanly possible—and she's written a couple of books on the subject, including *Mud, Snow, and Cyclocross: How 'Cross Took Over U.S. Cycling* and *Saddle, Sore: A Women-Only Guide for You and Your Bike.*

Currently, she spends her time on the road, going from race to race and looking for the best stories while traveling with her boyfriend, cycling coach Peter Glassford—one of the experts in this book! One of the only hardships of so much travel is less time spent in the kitchen, but luckily, she enjoys writing about food almost as much as eating it. Follow along on her adventures on Twitter or Instagram via @mollyjhurford.

**Nanci Guest, MSc, RD, CSCS,** is a 2016 PhD candidate in nutritional sciences at the University of Toronto. Guest is an international sports nutrition consultant for Olympians as well as professional athletes and teams, including those in the NHL and CFL. She was the lead dietitian at both the 2010 Winter Olympics in Vancouver and the 2015 Pan Am and Parapan Am games in Toronto and the main nutrition consultant to more than 100 Russian athletes preparing for the 2014 Winter Olympics in Sochi. Guest has had numerous appearances on TV and radio shows, in print media, and at speaking engagements for sport health care professionals, coaches, and teams.